INTER FASTING FOR WOMEN AND AUTOPHAGY: 2 manuscripts

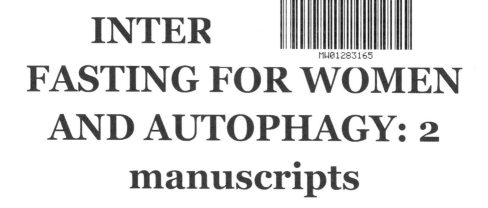

-

UNLOCKING THE SECRETS OF ANTI AGING AND EXTREME WEIGHT LOSS:

heal your body, burn fat, and reset your metabolism with this metabolic guide

By Serena Baker

Additionally, the information in the following pages is intended only for informational purposes and should thus be thought of as universal. As befitting its nature, it is presented without assurance regarding its prolonged validity or interim quality. Trademarks that are mentioned are done without written consent and can in no way be considered an endorsement from the trademark holder.

TABLE OF CONTENTS

Autophagy Book 11

Introduction 13
Chapter 1: Understanding Autophagy 15
Ch 1.1: The What and How of Autophagy 17

Functions of Autophagy 25

Ch 1.2: Variations of Autophagy 28

Macro-autophagy 29
Micro-autophagy 31
Chaperone-mediated Autophagy (CMA) 31

Ch 1.3: Benefits on the Cells, Body, and More 33
Ch 1.4: Risks and Cautions of Performance Autophagy 37
Ch 1.5: Detoxing: The Side Effects 41

Important, Helpful Guidelines During a Detox 42

Chapter 2: Activating Autophagy 44

Ch 2.1: Ways to Initiate Autophagy 47

Exercise 47
Ketosis 48
Fasting 48
Intermittent Water Fasting 49

Ch 2.2: Exercise 50
Ch 2.3: Ketosis 59

Insulin and Ketosis 62

Ch 2.4: Fasting 68
Ch 2.5: Intermittent Water Fasting 72

Chapter 3: Autophagy Performance 74

Ch 3.1: Ketosis Diets 76
Ch 3.2: Steps to Water Fasting 83
Ch 3.3: Weight Loss and Water Fasting 88

Ch 3.4: Muscle Mass and Water Fasting 90
Ch 3.5: Extended Water Fasting 92

Chapter 4: Optimizing Autophagy 93

Ch 4.1: Right Diet 95
Ch 4.2: Right Exercise 103
Ch 4.3: Right Fasting 107
Ch 4.4: Right Resting 111

Chapter 5: Autophagy for Everyone 114

Ch 5.1: Frequently Asked Questions (Regarding Autophagy, Ketosis, and Fasting) 115
Ch 5.2: Myths About Autophagy 118
Ch 5.3: Testimonials 121

Conclusion 123
Image Bibliography 124

Intermittent Fasting for Women Book 125

Introduction 129
Chapter 1: Intermittent Fasting for Men vs. Women 132

The Science of the Human Body 133
Reasons for Sex Distinction with IF 136

Chapter 2: Intermittent Fasting as a Woman 138

Hormones & Health: Weight Loss 138
IF & the Female Body 139
Physical Effects of IF for Women 141
Using IF to Help with Periods, Fertility, and Metabolism 142

Chapter 3: Diet & Intermittent Fasting 144

Pros & Cons of IF as a Dietary/Lifestyle Choice 145
What Foods & Liquids Do 148
Managing Hunger & Other Useful Tips 151

Chapter 4: When to Avoid Intermittent Fasting as a Woman 154

Exploring the Pregnant Candidate 155
Exploring the Underweight Candidate 156
Exploring the Candidate with an Eating Disorder 157
Exploring the Diabetic Candidate 158
Exploring Problematic Character Traits 159

Chapter 5: Different Methods of Intermittent Fasting 162

Crescendo Method 163
Lean-Gains Method (14:10) 164
16:8 Method 165
20:4 Method 165
12:12 Method 166
5:2 Method 167
Eat-Stop-Eat (24 Hour) Method 168
Alternate-Day Method 169
The Warrior Method 170
Spontaneous Skipping Method 171
Which Method Suits Which Woman & Which Lifestyle Best 172

Chapter 6: How to Get Started 175

Transitional Tips 176
Help for Routine-Setting 177
What to Expect 178
What to Do/What Not to Do 181
What to Lookout For 182
When to Quit 183
Most Common Mistakes & How to Avoid Them 184
Protecting Against Potential Roadblocks & Hiccups 186

Chapter 7: Intermittent Fasting for the Overworked & Stressed-Out Woman 188

IF & Its Effects on Stress 189
How to Start Without Adding More Stress 190
Best Foods & Drinks to Incorporate 191
Best Fasting Method for You 195

Chapter 8: Intermittent Fasting for the Breastfeeding Woman 197

The Arguments in the Field: A Good Idea or Not? 198
Possible Dangers 200
What Methods Have Worked 201
Eating Right While Breastfeeding 204

Chapter 9: Intermittent Fasting for the Woman with PCOS 217

What Is PCOS? 218
How IF Helps with PCOS 218
Best Foods & Diets for PCOS 219
Best Treatments & Exercises for PCOS 222
Best (IF) Tips on How to Lose Weight for PCOS 226

Chapter 10: Intermittent Fasting for the Mature or Menopausal Woman 229

Differences Between the Young vs. Older Woman 229
How IF Affects Women at This Age & How to Approach It 231
Anti-Aging Foods 232
Tips & Exercises to Lose Belly Fat & Kickstart Your Metabolism 236
Best (IF) Methods for Health & Weight Loss at This Age 237

Chapter 11: Autophagy & Intermittent Fasting for Women 239

What Is Autophagy? What Is Protein Cycling? 239
Autophagy, Protein Cycling, and Women's Health 240
How IF Affects People (concerning to Autophagy) 241

Chapter 12: 12 Useful Recipes for Weight Loss with Intermittent Fasting 243

Breakfast Recipes 243

Yogurt with Berries & Chia Seeds 243
DIY Omelet for Your Needs 245

Lunch Recipes 247

Fish Tacos with Lemon Dill Slaw 247
Late-Summer Salad 249
Tri-Color Potato & Black Bean Hash 251

Snack Recipes 253

Homemade Trail Mix 253
Homemade Grainy (Avocado) Toast 255

Dinner Recipes 258

Salmon with Wild Rice & Greens 258
Hearty Vegetable Stew 260
Chicken Breast with Grilled & Raw Vegetables 263

Dessert Recipes 265

Low-Fat Blueberry Crumble 265
IF-Friendly Brownies 267

Conclusion 269

Autophagy:

Live healthy. Discover your self-cleansing body's natural intelligence! Activate the anti-aging process through the ketosis state, extended water, intermittent fasting, and ketogenic diet!

By Serena Baker

Introduction

The human body is a vast universe of intelligence. We often forget how sophisticated our internal machinery is, and our daily lives were spent focusing on the external results. So much of our life-long health is determined by what goes on inside on a microscopic level. What you cannot see going on inside of you is immense. Every meal you eat, every beverage you drink, and every moment of rest or exertion have a lasting impact on your internal machinery.

All of us are looking for the right diet, exercise routine, and prescription drug to make us look and feel good for all of our lives. We sport the latest fad diet, intending to get healthier, energized, or lose weight, and we concentrate only on our fitness regimens as our way of supporting a long, healthy life, free of disease and chronic illness. All of these things contribute to something much deeper. With the right intake of food, exercise, and an occasional break from both, your body begins to experience autophagy.

Over time, our cells produce by-products and waste from the hard work that they are constantly doing. This microscopic bio-waste is collected in the cell, like an overflowing trash can. This happens when we eat too many sugars and carbohydrates, changing our insulin absorption and affecting our whole system's ability to function properly. When the cells are running slow because the waste is building up on account of a poor diet, lack of exercise, and our over-consumption of food daily, slowly over time, we begin to see the results: cancer, diabetes, inflammatory disease, cardiovascular disease, and rapid aging.
Our bodies are intelligent and know how to clean house and heal, especially if we create the right conditions for this process to occur. Autophagy is a self-healing mechanism at the cellular

level that when achieved can change the health of your whole life. This book is an instruction manual, giving you guidance about what it is and how it works, why and when to activate it, and what results you can expect from autophagy performance. Your health is in your hands all the way down to your cells. Begin your healing journey now!

Chapter 1: Understanding Autophagy

You may already have a basic understanding on the way the body works—blood, muscles, and bones—operated by a computer called the brain that sends information throughout the body to allow it to operate. We have systems for everything: digestion, breathing, going to the bathroom, and reproducing. Every part of us is a system, and those systems are built with cells. The basic building block of every person starts with a tiny, little machine with its own set of rules and orders.

In order to understand autophagy, you must consider the cell and how trillions of them create your everyday being. They all function individually, as part of a whole system and finally as a whole working human body. Like all living things, there are types of organisms that we all have inside of us, like microbes, bacteria, free radicals, and viruses that cannot function unless all of our cells are running on a healthy level. Some of these things such as microbes and certain bacteria are good and wanted in the system, while other forms of bacteria, free radicals, and viruses are what we want our cells to fight off and destroy. How can our cells effectively fight anything if they are unhealthy?

Fighting against all of the illnesses, diseases, inflammations, and other concerns of our health is the work of the cell. Right now, in our society, there is a huge lack of understanding about how we all give ourselves the toxins and poisons that create cell dysfunction, that leads to illness and loss of life. The reason why we all have diseases is because we are giving it to ourselves, through our foods, drinks, lack of exercise, processed foods, chemicals, and pollution.

If you want a healthy, long life, you have to understand the internal partnership of your cells and your overall well-being. It's not a matter of what drug you can take to fix the problem quickly, or what surgery can be performed to extract disease. Health and wellness begin inside, on a deep, cellular level. We cannot expect to feel well if we do not heal from this microscopic point of view. The chronic plague of cancer, diabetes, neurodegenerative illnesses, and all the inflammatory disorders and dysfunctions come from one, significant point: the health of the cell.

There are reasons for poor health and poor physical performance that stem from the ability or lack of ability for your cells to clean themselves or eat-away at the biowaste that comes naturally to a hard-working organism. This ability is autophagy. Autophagy is very simply put as cell function. It is a normal occurrence that allows for the proper recycling of material. There are specific functions in every cell, based on what part of the body or system they operate in. Some are muscle cells, others make up your brain, while several are responsible for the building up and breaking down of bone.

We don't behave in our lives, thinking about how and what we do to affect these tiny, little parts of us. We tend to view life from the macroscopic point of view; it is in our nature to do so. There is so much occurring every moment that we cannot see or feel. Knowing and understanding how our bodies function at a cellular level is the key to healing ourselves.

Beginning your course in understanding autophagy starts with the basics. To know autophagy, you have to know the cell and how it functions.

Ch 1.1: The What and How of Autophagy

Autophagy, when broken down, translates from Greek to mean "self-eating." This is a normal, biological process in the human body that occurs on the cellular level, deep within the cytoplasm. Breaking down the cell and its components can shed more light on why autophagy occurs in the first place.

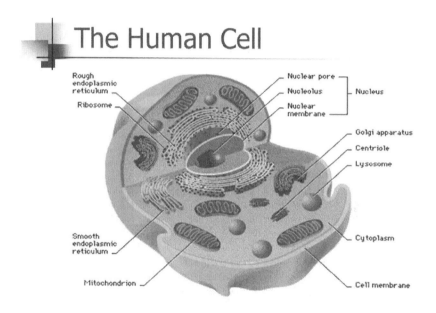

The basic cell of any human is made of proteins, lipids, cholesterol, and water, and these components make up the mechanisms that encourage healthy cell performance.

A cell is a sophisticated machine comprised of many organelles, plasma, amino acids, glucose, genetic information, and chemical compounds that help the cell to perform its functions. Here is a breakdown of what you will find within every cell in the body, no matter what body system it is working in:

Nucleus

- The nucleus has a double membrane and is a spherical shape containing your DNA strands. This part of the cells dictates protein synthesis, playing a major role in our cell performance, most specifically active transport of genetic information, metabolism, growth, and heredity.

Nucleoli

- A dense region, and part of the nucleus, the nucleoli play a major part in the creation of ribosomes.

Ribosome

- Tiny particles in the cell made of rRNA sub-particles. The job of the ribosome is to synthesize proteins. It is often referred to as the protein factory of the cell.

Cilia

- These are short, hair-like extensions on the outer surface of the cell that can move substances or particles over the outer surface.

Plasma Membrane

- This is the phospholipid layer of the skin of the cell. It is studded with proteins and serves as the cell's gatekeeper, the castle wall. When there are carbohydrates and proteins on the outer side of the cell, they will perform certain functions connected to the plasma membrane such as allowing for individual cell identification as a receptor for certain hormones, like the gatekeepers at the gate.

Mitochondria

- This organelle is a network of membranous folds covered in enzymes and is where your ATP, or adenosine triphosphate, is synthesized. They are referred to as the cell powerhouses, creating energy on the microscopic level for the whole body.

Lysosomes

- A round, bubble-like organelle, covered in a membrane, the lysosome is the digestive system or recycling center of the cell.

Centrioles

- A pair of hollow cylinders made up of tiny tubules, the function of the centriole is cell reproduction.

Golgi Apparatus

- A stack of flat, membranous sacs, the Golgi apparatus chemically processes and packages substances from the endoplasmic reticulum.

Endoplasmic Reticulum (ER)

- There is rough ER and smooth ER. Rough ER is covered in ribosomes, while smooth ER has no attached organelles. The ER is a network of sacs and canals and has a membranous quality.

Every human cell performs certain functions. Some functions of the cell are to maintain its own survival, and other functions are to maintain the body's survival. Most of the time, the number and type of organelles allow the cells to differ dramatically regarding how they specifically function. For example, cells that contain a large number of mitochondria, such as cardiovascular muscle cells, are capable of sustained work. The excess of mitochondria can synthesize more ATP to have more energy in the cell; they can support the necessary energy required for ongoing rhythmic contractions. Movement of the flagellum of sperm, the only cell in the body to have a flagellum (tail), is another example of a specialized organelle and its specific function. The sperm, a cell in the male reproductive system, is propelled by the flagellum through the reproductive tract of the female, increasing the chances of fertilization. Every cell has a distinct purpose and health.

All cells require some movement bringing things in and pushing things out. The movement of substances through cells is a major aspect of our ability to live healthfully. If our cells reject nutrient because they are unable to absorb any, then you and your cells will suffer.

The plasma membrane in a healthy cell separates the contents of the cell from the tissue fluid that surrounds it. At the same time, the membrane has to permit certain substances and chemical compounds to enter the cell and allow others to depart. Heavy traffic moves continuously in both directions through all cell membranes. Things like water molecules, food molecules, gases, wastes, and many others flow in and out of cells in an endless procession. There are two general ways this process occurs: *passive* and *active* transport processes.

Active transport requires the expenditure of energy by the cell; passive transport does not. The energy required for the active transport process is obtained through ATP or adenosine triphosphate. ATP is created in the mitochondria of the cell, using energy from nutrients, and is capable of releasing that energy to do work within the cell. For active transport to occur, the breakdown of ATP and use of that released energy are required.

The details of active and passive transport are much easier to understand if you remember two key facts:

1. Passive transport—no cellular energy is required to move substances from a high to a low concentration.

2. Active transport—cellular energy is required to move substances from a low to a high concentration.

Within each kind of transport, you can break it down further to understand the function of the cell and how it operates to stay healthy, and perform the various functions that work to keep the body alive. For example, within passive transport processes, there is diffusion, which includes osmosis and dialysis and filtration; within active transport processes, there is the ion pump, phagocytosis, and pinocytosis.

Active transport processes are what autophagy explains. Phagocytosis is most closely linked to the concept of autophagy. Autophagy is similar in that is the eating of materials within the cell. And like the transport processes, autophagy has its own variations that you will read about in the next chapter.

Bringing these concepts into a frame, consider the process of autophagy from the perspective of the lysosome.

The *lysosome* is the part of the cell to pay particular attention to when learning and understanding autophagy. It has the nickname "digestive bags" in some biological documents because of its particular job within the cell. They contain the enzymes that digest food substances. It isn't just food that they digest; they are also responsible for the digestion of microbes that invade the cell, and waste materials collected in the cell that need to be removed. Lysosomes protect the cell against destruction; they are also, in a way, the immune system of the cell.

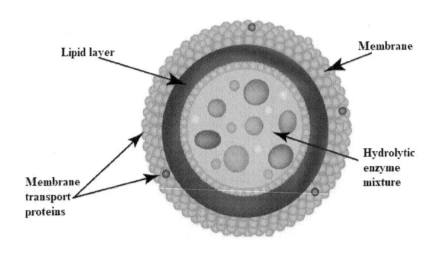

Lysosome

The lysosome searches for pieces and parts of old, worn down, and discarded cell material, such as dead organelles, damaged proteins, oxidized particles, and other bio-waste. The cells absorb the waste matter and collect useful components to build new cell parts. It is essentially your body's recycling system that occurs on a microscopic level. This process is what allows the body to eliminate faulty, errant organisms, a cancerous growth, and cell metabolism dysfunction.

Autophagy is not to be confused with apoptosis, which is the death of the entire cell. Apoptosis is normal and occurs as a part of cell growth and development. Autophagy is the removal of dead or dysfunctional bio-matter in the cell, some of which is recycled and repaired for future use, rather than overall death of the whole machine. It is the body's system for cleaning house.

Unlike our own digestive system, our cells cannot simply flush their waste down the toilet.

This process is also known to assist in your body's ability to have strong immunity and fight inflammation which can lead to a variety of health issues. Some inflammation is beneficial to your body, as when you are fighting a cold or healing from an acute wound, however, regular existence of inflammation in your body can break down your cellular function and lead to dysfunction. When you break it down, autophagy is our body's way of keeping us healthy, cancer-free, fit, energized, mentally well, and living longer. It is an adaptive response in the face of all stress.

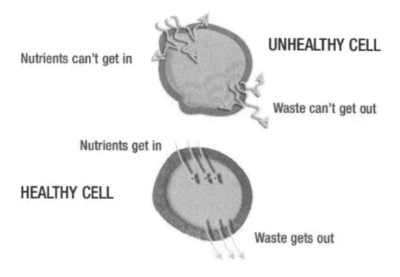

UNHEALTHY CELL

Nutrients can't get in

Waste can't get out

Nutrients get in

HEALTHY CELL

Waste gets out

When cells are stressed, such as lacking nutrients, energy, insulin, or become damaged from chronic variations of all of the above, a stress response occurs which initiates autophagy. It may seem counter-intuitive, but our cell's functioning improves when we are in a state of stress—healthy stress, of course.

What is healthy stress? Exercise, fasting, and ketosis. Without this kind of healthy stress, our cells will perform moderately and not optimally, suggesting that if you want to induce a serious, healing change in your body, you need to induce autophagy with the appropriate stress.

Autophagy is considered beneficial for many reasons, including the rejuvenation of the cells to impact life-long health and balance. When your cells age the machinery within, the cell also ages and becomes dysfunctional or nonfunctional. Autophagy is a biological maneuver to refresh and renew the cell by eliminating waste or recycling it for more efficient use and performance. By this method of cellular repair, the idea is that you can activate autophagy intentionally to promote cell rejuvenation that will reduce chances of certain age-related illnesses, diseases, and disorders. It can also repair existing conditions like diabetes, obesity, and food and health-related disorders that are the result of poor diet and lack of exercise. Several studies have shown improvement in neurodegenerative disorders, too, such as Parkinson's and Alzheimer's.

Think of it like the cell-cleansing garbage disposal crew. We have our own self-cleaning system when our cells are dirty with a build-up of old waste. It can represent in the way we feel and even the way we look. If you have dry, flaky skin and limp damaged hair, it may be due to the cell clutter that hasn't been able to clean for some reason. If you are fatigued, overweight, and aching all over, it may be because your cells cannot perform optimally under those conditions. Looking deeper into the cell will tell you more about the functions of autophagy.

Functions of Autophagy

Nutrient Starvation

Autophagy has roles in a variety of cellular functions. In yeasts, for example, the nutrient starvation activates a high level of autophagy. This permits unneeded proteins to be broken down and amino acids to be recycled for the synthesis of proteins that are necessary for survival. Autophagy is induced in higher eukaryotes in response to the nutrient depletion that occurs at birth when the trans-placental food supply is cut off, as well as that of nutrient-starved cultured cells and tissues. In nutrition-deficient conditions, Mutant yeast cells that have a reduced autophagic capability rapidly cease to be. Studies suggest that autophagy is indispensable for protein degradation in the vacuoles under fasting conditions and that around 15 APG genes are involved in autophagy in yeast. The gene ATG7 has been implicated in nutrient-mediated autophagy; starvation-induced autophagy was impaired in *atg7*-deficient mice.

Xenophagy

Xenophagy is the autophagic degradation of infectious particles. Our innate immunity is dependent upon our cellular autophagic machinery. Intracellular pathogens, like the bacterium which is responsible for tuberculosis, are chosen for degradation by the same cellular machinery and regulatory mechanisms that choose host mitochondria for mortification. This is further evidence for the endosymbiotic hypothesis, an evolutionary theory of origin. This process leads to the destruction of the invasive microorganisms; however, some bacteria can halt the maturing process of phagosomes. Activating autophagy help overcome infected cells, restoring pathogen degradation.

Infection

In the same family as the rabies virus, vesicular stomatitis virus is taken up by the autophagosome and translocated to the lysosomes, where detection of certain gene codes through a receptor occurs. After the activation of the receptor, intracellular signaling is initiated, inducing interferon and other antiviral cytokines. Viruses and bacteria subvert the autophagic pathway to promote their own replication. A protein known as Galectin-8 has recently been called an intracellular receptor for dangerous particles, capable of initiating autophagy to protect against intracellular pathogens. Galectin-8 binds to a damaged vacuole or organelle and then enlists an autophagy adaptor, leading to the formation of an autophagosome.

Repair

Autophagy deteriorates damaged cell matter such as oxidized proteins, damaged organelles, and another biowaste. Dysfunctional autophagy is considered one of the main reasons for the accumulation of damaged cells and aging.

Apoptosis

The appearance of autophagosomes can be an indicator of programmed cell death or apoptosis and depends on autophagy proteins. Autophagy is not the death of a cell; it is the renewal; however, within certain conditions, an internal cell death happens, and certain byproducts are collected and consumed. There has been confusion between apoptosis and cell and autophagy and whether they are linked. There has been a suggestion that autophagy causes cell death; however, autophagic performance in dying cells is actually an attempt to prevent the death of the cell.

Allowing your understanding of autophagy to form through all of the data and research can help you see the effect it has on almost all living things at all times. We are almost always in some state of autophagy on the cellular level; however, your cells may not be able to fully engage in the full-blown renewal of the cells that can help prevent disease and slow the aging process. The result of autophagy is that your cells get the deep-clean overhaul that they need to be renewed, refreshed and functioning full steam ahead. And the great thing is that you can activate autophagy through a few, simple steps, but before reading into the activation process, there is more to know about the various types of autophagy. In short, your healthy cells are actively autophagic, and your unhealthy cells are not.

Ch 1.2: Variations of Autophagy

Autophagy was originally noticed by Keith Porter and his student Thomas Ashford in January of 1962. Their reports showed an increased number of lysosomes in rat liver cells after the addition of glucagon. Some of the rats also showed displaced lysosomes near the center of the cell. Originally, they called this discovery autolysis. Unfortunately, Porter and Ashford wrongly interpreted the findings of their experiments as lysosome formation.

Shortly after in 1963, another group of scientists published a detailed description of what they called "focal cytoplasmic degradation," referencing a 1955 German study. The findings detailed three continuous stages of maturation of the cytoplasm to lysosomes. The process was thought to be limited to injury states that functioned under physiological conditions, leading to a rejuvenation of materials and disposal of wasted organelles.

Christian de Duve, a Belgian biochemist, was inspired by the research and decided to call it "autophagy," the Greek word for self-eating. He came up with the name as a part of the lysosomal function while explaining the role of glucagon as a major activator of cell degradation in the liver. He posited that lysosomes are responsible for autophagy. This was the first time that lysosomes were considered the site of intracellular autophagy.

Fast forward to the 1990s when several different groups of scientists discovered autophagy-related genes, independently of each other using the yeast growth for the experiments. Yoshinori Ohsumi and Michael Thumm examined starvation-induced non-selective autophagy, which led to a Pulitzer Prize for Ohsumi and his work in this subject. Another scientist, Daniel Klionsky uncovered the cytoplasm-to-vacuole targeting pathway, a form of selective autophagy. Eventually, they discovered that they were looking at the same pathway from different perspectives. The genes discovered by the yeast experiment groups were given a variety of names like APG, AUT, CVT, GSA, PAG, PAZ, and PDD. A unified name was decided by researchers, using ATG to denote autophagy genes. The 2016 Nobel Prize in Physiology or Medicine was awarded to Yoshinori Ohsumi for these findings. There has been accelerated growth in the study of autophagy since the early 2000s. Knowledge of ATG genes offered scientists better tools to understand the functions of autophagy in human health and disease. Autophagy and cancer were being closely studied, and there were landmark discoveries within certain research groups showing evidence of the cancer prevention quality of autophagy. Research in neurodegenerative health and auto-immune disease began to take off at this time as well. Since the blossoming of knowledge surrounding autophagy, the studies have continued to gain momentum, and evidence of its ability to heal is still being studied and researched as more and more people bring it into their daily health practices.

There are three main types of autophagy to know, and each one paints a more colorful picture about what is actually happening inside the cell. The three types are macro-autophagy, micro-autophagy, and chaperone-mediated autophagy.

Macro-autophagy

The cell is like a tiny city, comprised of various structures that are all whirring and wheeling to accomplish their inputs and outputs. An autophagosome is a membrane or vesicle in the cell that will fuse with lysosomes.

Autophagosomes form through a process by which omegasomes on the endoplasmic reticulum elongate and become phagophores. Through a communication on the cellular level through the genes Atg 12-Atg-5 and some other chemical complexes, the autophagosome forms and begins to evolve into a spherical shape, encapsulating any free-floating waste, carting it to the lysosome. Imagine Pac Man devouring power pellets. Once the waste material is fully enclosed in the newly formed autophagosome, it will make its way to the nearest lysosome in the cell.

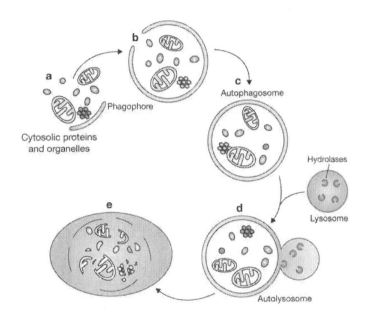

As the recycling plant, the lysosome is full of enzymes to transform waste matter into useful matter. The autophagosome makes contact with the membrane of the lysosome, and they fuse together, allowing the autophagosome to transfer the collected garbage to the recycling plant. Essentially, the autophagosome is the trash collector bringing a truckload of plastic and cardboard to the lysosome to get turned into useful materials.

Micro-autophagy

This process of autophagy is strikingly similar to macro-autophagy, the difference being that the lysosome does all the work. The waste materials are collected like Pac Man chomping pellets; however, in micro-autophagy, the lysosome does the encapsulating and eating. This organelle has the ability to receive waste from the passing autophagosome but can just as easily absorb the waste on its own, meaning that it works twice as hard to clean the cell of unnecessary debris.

The same process of transmutation occurs within the lysosome as it would in macro-autophagy, recycling matter for renewed used and better cell function.

Chaperone-mediated Autophagy (CMA)

With this type of autophagy, the process is much more selective. Unlike macro- and micro-autophagy in which the garbage man just goes around collecting trash, in CMA, there are specific orders and coordinates. It is a timed transfer or translocation of certain protein compounds that need extraction from their current location and guidance by a "chaperone" to the lysosome. CMA is more like a private army who receives orders that must be carried out.

Once you are able to identify the process by understanding the different ways autophagy can occur inside the cell, you can picture the process and connect the dots with why you might want to activate autophagy in your body. If you have never fasted, experienced ketosis through your food intake, or had any kind of exercise routine, then you are likely walking around with some very cluttered cells that need some serious cleanup. Autophagy is always happening on some level; however, when you are not creating circumstances to help it occur optimally, then it is only working at a moderate to low level of efficiency. There are many ways that initiating autophagy can improve your health and prevent serious or chronic health conditions later in life.

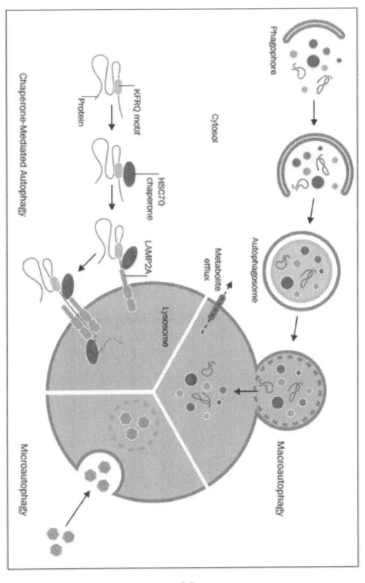

Ch 1.3: Benefits on the Cells, Body, and More

It is the preservation of life when the body is working to fight off something in times of stress or even starvation. This microscopic performance activates to repair the cells and any damage that could be caused by illness and inflammation. This process can also deplete or starve unwanted intruders from the vital nutrients they need to survive, allowing for their death and renewal.

The benefits of autophagy are limitless and can change your body function deep down on the cellular level. Some benefits are:

- *Promotion of a longer, healthier life through cell regeneration*

- *Helps in weight loss by encouraging healthier metabolism*—Autophagy can help clean and restore the toxic accumulation in the mitochondria, the energy makers of the cell. This is where fat gets burned and Adenosine Triphosphate (ATP) is produced. ATP is the compound that provides certain cellular energy, specifically muscle contraction. Autophagy allows for greater efficiency to boost metabolism and energy stores.

- *Risks of neurodegenerative disease are decreased*—Diseases in the brain take a long time to occur and happen over time with the buildup of misfolded, old, or dysfunctional proteins in or around the brain cells. The chemical compounds linked to the cause of Parkinson's disease, synuclein, is removed through autophagy. Studies suggest that the same may be true in cases of

Alzheimer's, removing the compound amyloid from the brain that is known to be associated with this disease. Another neurodegenerative disease is dementia caused by diabetes. Chronic insulin resistance disallows autophagy from occurring so no clean up can occur within the cell, leaving them in a toxic wasteland of malfunction.

- *Regulation of inflammation*—Autophagy allows inflammation when it is needed to fight off invaders, yet also reduces inflammation when it is the chronic response to over-triggered signals to the cells and the body.

- *Helps fight infectious disease*

- *Improves muscle performance*—Muscles undergo stress during exercise. Microscopic tearing in the fibers of muscles occurs during strenuous activity. The muscle fibers, also made of specific kinds of cells, are repaired through the process of autophagy. Over time, as you build muscle, it will reduce the amount of energy needed to utilize the muscle in general.

- *Prevents the onset of cancer*—Though research is still being done to understand the effects of autophagy on various kinds of cancer, studies have indicated that it can help to prevent cancer from forming. Scientists who have studied the impact of impaired autophagic response in mice see an up-rise of cancer in the mice. To perform the study, the mice involved had their autophagic response mechanism cut off from fully functioning. The result was cancer. The question is, can it work as a treatment for cancer, instead of just preventing it through autophagy? How would inducing autophagy impact other treatments?

More research must be done to understand the impact of induced autophagy in pre-existing cancer treatments like chemotherapy, but it may be that it could have a greater benefit than chemo which can be incredibly damaging to the body if applied long term.

- *Improvement in digestive health*—Autophagy is activated through fasting for short periods intermittently. The break from calorie intake and digestion alone can help your digestive system immensely; everyone needs a break now and then. More to that, while your body is resting from needing to digest, the cells that make up your digestive system and all other systems in your body will be activated to perform autophagy because of the fast, leading to a purification of the cells.

- *Improves the health of the skin*—Damage from sun exposure, toxins in the air, changes in temperature, acute ailments like bruises, scrapes, punctures, and burns may all benefit from the autophagic performance. While you may be constantly replacing cells, autophagy keeps the cells fresh and renewed, giving a glow to the skin.

- *Minimizes cell death or apoptosis*—With autophagy functioning, the cells are constantly being cleaned and rejuvenated; without it, the cells are piling up with waste and eventually struggle to perform well, leading to a programmed death of the cell. When that happens, the cell leaves behind trash that needs to be taken out, and if the cell itself is dead, autophagy won't occur because the process occurs inside the cell. The body will have to trigger an inflammatory response to clean up the cell death aftermath.

- *Improved cognition, memory, and brain function—* Autophagy enhances neuroplasticity, the brain's ability to form and reorganize synaptic connections. There is an increase in cognitive ability through the increase of mitochondria. When your brain cells can function well, so can your whole brain.

- *Regulation of hormones, which allows for overall body high performance and function.*

- *Improves cardiovascular health—*Autophagy works to clean toxins and biowaste from the cells of the heart muscle, which is constantly pumping blood through your whole body. Aiding in the general renewal of these cells brings about a better functioning heart.

The list goes on, and discoveries about the effects of autophagy on the health of the body continue to demonstrate the beneficial impact of the autophagic performance. When you create opportunities to enhance and promote autophagy, you are enhancing and promoting the health of every cell in your body.

Ch 1.4: Risks and Cautions of Performance Autophagy

Before you move ahead and begin the process of activating autophagy, it is important to be aware of cautions and risks. To have the best benefit from creating this healing response, you need to plan ahead and be informed about how to do it properly so that you don't cause yourself harm.

There are three main ways that you will learn to activate autophagy in this book: exercise, ketosis, and fasting. When covering the risks, you will understand what can happen or potentially go wrong while using these methods to activate autophagy. Bear in mind that if you are suffering from any severe medical issues, chronic illness, or disease, then it is always a good idea to consult a doctor before beginning this process.

This chapter will briefly cover some of the risks and precautions in initiating autophagy so that you can be prepared to plan your experience well. The next chapters in the book will go into greater detail about each method of activating autophagy.
Some risks and precautions:

- *Losing the wrong kind of weight*—If you lose muscle instead of fat, you are losing the wrong kind of weight. If you don't need to lose a lot of fat through diet, or fasting, then you have to ensure that you consume enough fat prior to fasting. Your body must be prepared to enter a period without calorie intake, and if you have no fat to burn, then you may find yourself losing some muscle. This is not usually the case if you are fasting properly, preparing in advance, and giving your body time to rest while you are on the fast. Some people will try to do intense exercise on a fast to create an even greater increase in the autophagic response. This is when your body will start to turn to the protein of your body for energy. Make sure you are approaching fasting to induce autophagy healthily.

- *Dehydration*—During an intermittent water fast, you may run the risk of dehydration. Fasting is taking a break from food and food contains a percentage of your daily water intake. You will need to make sure you are drinking the right amount of water to stay hydrated. On the other hand, drinking too much water can drown the cells, and drinking too much, too fast can lead to hyponatremia which is the loss of sodium in the body. Loss of salt in your body can lead to an extreme drop in blood pressure. Drop in sodium levels due to excess water will cause fluid shifts from outside to inside the cell. The swell causes pressure in the skull which can lead to headache, nausea, and vomiting. Severe cases of decreased blood pressure can lead to confusion, problems breathing, sleepiness, confused state, weakened muscles, and cramping.

- *Urge to overeat after fasting*—Returning to food after a fast must be done slowly, in steps. When you are not healthily performing a fast, you may be inclined to overeat following the fasting period. If done regularly, this can have a detrimental impact on the body, causing shock to your system.

- *Extreme fasting can lead to starvation and eventually death*

- *If you fast for too long your body will start to eat itself—* If you are performing a fast for an extreme length of time without any calories, or supplements, your body will start to eat muscle, including cardiovascular muscle and also cells like brain cells. This can be avoided by choosing the right length of time for your fast, the right fast for your needs, and the right mineral and vitamin supplement to aid the process and prevent muscle loss. There is an important window of benefit for creating autophagy in a fast—between activation and the point where your body stops burning fat and starts eating muscle.

- *Loss of vitamins and minerals from food can cause health problems*—It is important to allow a mineral supplement. Since there are no calories in many supplements, you will not be breaking the fast, although some vitamins can cause discomfort in the stomach if not taken with food, so finding the right vitamins is important for fasting comfort.

- *Less serious, but important precautions and risks is the effect on mood*—Irritability, moodiness, highs and lows, energy depletion, low blood pressure, and dizziness.

- *Improper fasting can raise stress hormone levels*- If you are not engaging in fasting properly, you may encounter the issue of increased stress hormones in the body which isn't good for long periods, and can be very damaging to many systems.

- *Fast detoxifying can impact your health*—The rate of detox when fasting is rapid. Toxins held in your body fat for long periods will release in your bloodstream as your body burns fat for calorie consumption. Too many toxins in the bloodstream can feel terrible and lead to nausea, sickness, and a general unwell feeling.

- *A fasting high can impact your cognitive ability*— Sometimes during a fast, you may experience fasting high, a feeling of euphoria as your body shifts and heals. Sometimes, this mental state can make it challenging for you to reasonably listen to your body, making sure you are not overdoing it.

A majority of the risks and precautions can be easily avoided if you approach autophagic performance with knowledge and preparation. Because the benefits of autophagy are so powerful, it is worth experiencing. With the right diet, exercise, fasting, and rest, you can healthfully activate autophagy safely and beneficially.

Ch 1.5: Detoxing: The Side Effects

Detoxing is simply your body's process for eliminating toxins. Unlike autophagy which works on the cellular level to eat wastes and toxins to turn them into something better, detoxing requires removal through the bloodstream, skin (sweat, rashes, outbreaks) and excrement or urine. Detoxing can occur through switching to certain diets, specifically designed for detox results, fasting, and exercise.

There are many side effects to detoxing which is why taking care to do it gently and responsibly will allow for a healthier experience overall. Some of the symptoms of detoxing are:

- Skin breakouts in various places

- Body aches and spasms

- Digestive issues (flatulence, bloating, constipation, diarrhea)

- Mood swings

- Mental fog, low cognitive function

- Headache

- Crankiness and irritability

- Flu-like feeling

- Sleep issues

Inflammation from toxins in your body is what causes the symptoms as they are being released. Two to three days of discomfort can occur, depending on the individual, and especially if you are not accustomed to detoxing or have never done it before. Once symptoms clear, there is a feeling of mental clarity, energy, and renewal.

Important, Helpful Guidelines During a Detox

As you eliminate toxins by removing foods slowly into a fasting period, you can support and ease the transition in your body by following these steps:

- Coordinate your primary detox during a time when you can rest, like a weekend, holiday, or scheduled time when you are not working or have any major social plans.

- Eat healthy fats to support your transition and prevent extreme cravings, headaches, and fatigue.

- Drink extra water to help flush toxins from the system.

- Use sweating as well as water consumption to help eliminate toxins through the skin (steam shower, sauna, hot bath).

- Include fiber in your detox diet to eliminate smoothly and avoid constipation.

- Supplement with vitamins and minerals to support muscles, bones, joints, and tissues to prevent achiness, such as magnesium.

- Exercise to help activate detox through blood flow and sweating.

- Get plenty of rest and sleep.

- Include protein in your diet to keep blood sugar balanced (fish, beans, lean poultry, nuts, and seeds).

Symptoms and side effects of detoxing are a good sign that your body is working to eliminate the toxins you are carrying around. Treat yourself well, so you can get to the fasting stage that allows autophagy to work on the cellular level to help detoxify the cells, throughout the entire body.

Chapter 2: Activating Autophagy

This book isn't just about autophagy and what it is from a scientific or biological perspective. The purpose of this book is to show you how you can gain awareness of your own body intelligence to activate the power of your healing ability. It is amazing that we all carry this wisdom deep within our cells, yet most people have no knowledge of this process or why it is important to create opportunities for increased autophagy.

Once you understand the methods for activating autophagy, it is easy to consider bringing it into the fold of your regular diet, exercise, and lifestyle. If you have the knowledge to heal yourself, what would stop you?

So many people are surprised at the idea that we have the mechanisms to prevent and heal our illnesses and diseases. How we have spent the past hundred years, or so, is a direct link to the areas of our history that need attention. Not all science is fact. Some research has come and gone, having been disproven by new discoveries. We see it as a line in the sand when a group of researchers determine something new about long-held wisdom in the medical community. Crossing into the health lines of all, the research shows that one thing hasn't changed in our history as human beings, and that is our cellular design.

The basis of our survival across centuries hasn't come from the fad diet or the present-day version of correct exercise; we all have the understanding deep within us to prevent disease, and yet we can't help but struggle with the reality that men and women across the world are suffering from diseases. If you consider the ancient civilizations of men and women who foraged and hunted, you see that there wasn't any evidence of these illnesses. People might have had incurable ailments or severe injuries that caused an early death; however, cancer was not something detected in any archeological findings of human remains.

Piecing together the common denominators, what do we find? Serious illness isn't all inside us; it comes from everywhere outside of us—our choice of hamburgers and frozen pizza over kale and apples, our addiction to over-the-counter medications that only help you endure the symptoms but not cure the cause, our desire to relax on the couch with a TV show and stay inside with our cell phones, rather than go out for an evening stroll and enjoy the weather. All of these factors are outside of our bodies, and we are the one deciding to create these serious illnesses.

Facing the reality that you are causing your own illness isn't easy for anyone, and letting go of the sugar addictions, coffee habits, and favorite snack foods between meals has its challenges when your body is used to being fed these chemicals regularly.

What you can do to heal yourself is easy; all it takes is an eagerness to try. Because we have the internal body intelligence to heal, we need to know how to allow for that healing to begin. Thanks to the benefits of creating autophagy in our cells, we can now see what it is that is really kicking us into a position of cleansing and renewal.

There are several ways to activate this self-eating/self-healing process. A few of them all together prove to be most beneficial, allowing for a balanced, autophagic occurrence. When you start to ignite the process, you will understand the connection between each method of activation and how the healthier approach to stabilizing an autophagic detox will utilize several ways together. Like the cogs and wheels all working together to tell time.

Understanding each method separately will allow for a more fine-tuned, intentional approach to autophagy. It is important when activating this method of deep cellular healing that you attend to it carefully and healthily. Electing to use each method during your intentional autophagic activation, will provide you with the best results for internal repair and deep healing.

This chapter will approach each method and explain the how and why of each method as a source of autophagic initiation. Further chapters in this book will give more step by step guidance on performing these methods for increased autophagy.

Ch 2.1: Ways to Initiate Autophagy

There are multiple ways by which autophagy is activated in both plants and animals that occur in the natural world without design or purposeful initiation. When your body is operating optimally, autophagy is occurring optimally also. In our current culture, the air we breathe, the water we drink, the multiple meals a day full of carbs, sugars, stimulants, and highly processed materials default our bodies to a setting of low performance. The elegant autophagic dance within cannot occur properly under such conditions, and in order to return to balanced levels of regularly occurring autophagy in our cells, we must begin by initiating the process and using the methods of activation to assist our bodies in healthy cell regeneration.

Before you get started with preparing to activate autophagy intentionally, it is important to understand how and why the methods outlined in this chapter work to promote that process. The major methods that will be discussed and detailed in this chapter are exercise, ketosis fasting, and intermittent water fasting.

Exercise

The benefits of exercise are long proven to establish a healthy, balanced body. The effects of exercise on all systems of the body are profound, and autophagy is part of the reason for this. The stress you put on your muscles when you exercise brings about the activation of autophagy. There are a variety of ways to exercise, and some of them create a deeper impact on the cellular level than others. Exercise is also a large part of a smooth detoxification process. When you exercise, you increase your heart rate which pushes more fresh, oxygenated blood at a faster rate through your body, allowing for a swifter push and release of toxins coming out through a fasting or detox process, kind of like flushing the toilet.

With certain kinds of exercise, you can create a more impactful autophagic response, and coupled with some of the other methods, you bring about greater change and more abundant cell regeneration, upwards of 300% from if you weren't exercising at all, according to some research.

Ketosis

The process by which the body relies on fat stores for energy rather than sugars and carbohydrates is known as ketosis. More specifically, when certain foods are eliminated from the diet, the body turns to stored fats to burn as fuel. When the fat is used as energy, acids are left behind in the blood and are eliminated in the urine. These acids are known as ketones and are the indicator that you need to assure that fat is being burned.

Restricting calories in the diet and eliminating certain foods such as carbohydrates and sugars that turn into glucose, can stimulate the autophagic process by bringing about the change in cells through diet and ketosis.

Fasting

Fasting hasn't lost its mainstream impact since the dawn of early humans who scavenged the Earth for food. As we evolve, we can connect the dots more and more about certain methods of health and healing and the correlation with our early ancestors. Refraining from and restricting certain foods and eliminating them altogether, create an internal survival gateway to boost your body's need to stay alive until your next meal.

This connection to autophagy is what truly eliminates the wastes and toxins. As your diet becomes less involved, fewer meals and longer time between them, you instigate the action of cell renewal throughout the body systems. When you disengage from food for fuel, your body can rely on fat for fuel and give your cells an opportunity to clean house, so to speak.

Positive performance autophagy requires initiation through some food elimination and fasting. There are healthy methods and approaches as well as risks and dangers, so it will be important to have a handle on proper fasting methods before jumping in.

Intermittent Water Fasting

Along the history of humankind's search for food in times of foraging and hunting, at times, the only thing available was water. In today's health news, everyone insists on 8 glasses of water as the essential minimum requirement. The internal essence of every part of you, every muscle, organ, fiber, and cell, is water.

What you gain from fasting from food is an activation of autophagy; the goal of which is to recycle cell waste and rejuvenate the body from the cellular level. What you lose in the fasting process is water. Upwards of 30% of your daily water intake comes from food. When you take food away, you replace it with water. That is the basis of water fasting.

Intermittency is the timing of fasting for healthy, balanced autophagic performance. It will obviously cause irreparable damage to the body if you fast too long, too frequently. Fasting for short term periods is a healthy way to reestablish cellular function, and should be done alternating between eating a healthy diet and igniting autophagy with fasting.

As you can see, each method has its value and purpose in initiating autophagy. Together, these methods bring about cell renewal and regeneration, elimination of toxins, and prevention of disease. In the next sub-chapters, we will dig deeper into each method, assuring that you can healthily support autophagy for healing the cells.

Ch 2.2: Exercise

What happens to your body when you exercise? The answer lies on a deep, cellular level, not just in the physical results. Since early human existence, we have had to adapt and perform using our bodies to leverage the entire experience. Our bones, muscles, and tissues are what support us, keep us upright, and help us handle all activities in our everyday lives. Regardless of whether you are a caveman or a bank teller, you are using your muscles, bones, joints, and tissues, all of which are made up of tiny cells, specifically designed to function for each body process.

Early man had a greater need and opportunity to have regular exercise; it was the only way to survive. Before the advent of automobiles, factories, industry, and technology, human beings were required to use their bodies all the time, every day to accomplish the ins and outs of human existence. An exercise wasn't something you had to plan or schedule. Gym memberships were not a necessary part of reality. Life was exercise unless you were royalty and could lay around all day and eat decadent food to your heart's content, or rather discontent.

To understand the need for exercise on your body, you must look deep within the muscles and understand them on a cellular level. Bringing into focus the structure and function of your muscles, will bring you closer to understanding how autophagy can have an impact on this system, and why you want to create autophagy to heal this part of yourself.

Muscle is considered a soft tissue. It is found in most animals. Muscle cells are made of protein filaments that contain actin and myosin. These protein filaments glide past one another, creating contractions that change the length and the shape of the cell. Think of a bulging bicep: the muscle fibers collectively bulge to produce that shape when a certain action occurs. Force and motion are the functions of muscles. They have many roles such as moving your body in various ways, posture, internal organ movements like a heartbeat, and peristalsis, which is the movement of the digestive organs to move food through the body.

Myogenesis is the process by which the mesodermal layer of embryonic cells creates muscle tissue. The muscles can be divided into three types: striated (skeletal), smooth, and cardiac. The action of the muscle is either voluntary or involuntary. Involuntary muscles do not require conscious thought to function; they just perform their tasks, and you don't even realize it. The beat of the heart in cardiac muscle and the peristalsis of the intestines are examples of involuntary muscle movement. Skeletal or striated muscled requires conscious thought to move and is therefore called voluntary muscle movement. There are fast and slow twitch fibers when talking about skeletal muscle.

Oxidation of fats and carbohydrates is what powers muscles to make them move. Fast twitch fibers in skeletal muscles also use anaerobic chemical reactions. The reactions of the chemicals are what produced ATP, and adenosine triphosphate is what gives energy to the movement of the myosin heads in the muscle fibers.

The epimysium is a layer of tough connective tissue that sheaths the skeletal muscles. This tough tissue is what pins down the muscle tissues to the tendons. Bundles of fascicles lie within the epimysium, each one containing anywhere from 10 to 100 or more muscle fibers, all sheathed by another layer of tissue called perimysium. The perimysium is a pathway for nerves and blood flow to your muscles. Myocytes are the muscle cells and are like bundles of threads, encapsulated in its own collagenous endomysium tissue. The overall muscle is made up of all these tiny fibers that are all bundled together in fascicles to form your muscles. Every muscle is built of muscle cells.

Muscle function is supported by the membranes that surround each bundle, giving the energy and stamina it needs to resist passive stretching and maintain active performance.

Each muscle cell contains myofibrils. These are also bundled protein filaments and are complex strands of a variety of filaments that form to create sarcomeres. Sarcomeres are like candy canes, striated due to the intermittent layout of the skeletal and cardiac muscle. Actin and myosin are the filament components of the sarcomere.

There are significant differences between the three types of muscle, yet they all have the same cell function provided by the actin and myosin. The actin and myosin are what create the contraction of the muscle on the cellular level. The contraction of skeletal muscle on the cellular level is controlled by nerves that send electrical impulses from the brain, specifically, motoneurons (also cells). There are internal, pacemaker cells that are responsible for the involuntary movement of the cardiac and smooth muscles. The chemical neurotransmitter acetylcholine is what facilitates all skeletal and most smooth muscle contraction.

Movement of almost every muscle is decided by the origin and insertion of that muscle: where it comes from and what it attaches to. However, many sarcomeres are able to operate in a cross section of muscle determines the amount of force it can generate; the bigger your muscles, the thicker the sarcomeres, the greater the force. Every skeletal muscle is made of myofibrils, each one a chain of sarcomeres. The muscle cell contracts as one unit of sarcomeres, shortening simultaneously and lengthening simultaneously.

Leverage mechanics determines the amount of force that can occur in the action of the muscles in the external environment. An example of this would be flexing your biceps muscle.

Much of the body's energy consumption is through the movement of your muscles. Every muscle cell produces ATP which is the energy compound that creates the power to move the myosin heads in every muscle fiber. There is a short-term store of energy know as creatine phosphate, and it is born from the ATP. It can also regenerate ATP when it is needed with the compound known as creatine kinase. Muscles will also keep a store of glycogen, which is a form of glucose. It can be quickly turned into glucose when there is a need for sustained energy during incredibly powerful muscle contractions.

The molecule of glucose can be broken down anaerobically during glycolysis. Out of glycolysis 2 ATP and 2 lactic acid molecules are formed; however, this outcome is not produced in the aerobic state. Each muscle cell also has fat molecules that are utilized as energy during aerobic exercise. It takes longer to produce ATP in aerobic energy systems and requires more involved steps, yet it produces a great deal more ATP than what is seen in anaerobic glycolysis.

On another note, cardiac muscle can regularly consume all of the macronutrients listed above: protein, glucose, and fat. It can do this aerobically, as it is always working and pumping blood throughout the body. Also, the cardiac muscle will always take out the maximum amount of ATP from any involved molecule.

These muscle fibers, as well as the liver and red blood cells, often consume lactic acid that is usually put out by the skeletal muscles during exercise; in essence, exercise helps the cells of your heart function.

Human muscle efficiency has been measured at up to 18-26%. This ratio comes from a breakdown of the output of mechanical work against the total metabolism, calculated from the consumption of oxygen. Low efficiency comes from a lowered generation of ATP from your food energy intake, and also the loss of converting ATP into mechanical action within the muscle fibers, as well as overall mechanical loss within the body. The loss of efficiency depends on the type of exercise being performed and the type of muscle fibers being used.

Having an understanding of the cellular function of muscles is vital when you are considering the way autophagy works. To break it down, muscle is the result of three, important things:

1. Physiological strength = size of the muscle, cross section of muscle, response to training

2. Neurological strength = the strength of signal given to the muscles telling them to contract (strong or weak signal)

3. Mechanical strength = force, leverage, joint capability

Discovering the lessons within the cells brings you face to face with the commitment, to knowing the inner workings of the cell's ability to not only perform their functions but also their ability to heal. The fine tuning that occurs deep within comes from the sophisticated machinery that makes up your entire being: the cell. Muscle cells are as in need of autophagy as any other part of your body. Your muscles are your body, and if your muscle cells are unable to renew, then you lose the quality of function that keeps you feeling young and agile.

The vitality of out muscle health begins in the cell, like with all other systems in the body. One of the significant ways to activate autophagy is through the exercise of the muscles. Seeing the muscle up close helps you understand what is happening deep within when you exercise. The cells need cleansing so that your body can perform optimally. If you never exercise, how can your muscle cells do the work they are intended to do?

As we have engineered ways to unload the burden of labor onto machines and technology, we have accrued a need to find our daily dose of exercise in other ways. Many people have given up on exercise altogether, living in a culture that promotes a sedentary lifestyle in front of a TV, or a need to work for 8 hours straight sitting at a computer.

Our bodies need exercise to function well, and this has been proven over and over again. Benefits of exercise are far-reaching and here are a few examples:

- *Good for muscles and bones*—building and maintenance and the release of hormones to absorb amino acids in muscle and bone.

- *Increased energy levels*

- *Reduced risk of chronic disease*—improved insulin use, reduction of belly fat which leads to Type II diabetes, improved cardiovascular health, hormonal balance, oxygen-rich blood to improve the vital function of all body systems.

- *Weight loss*—there are three ways to lose weight: digestion, body functions like breathing and heartbeat, and exercise. Exercise increases your metabolism and when combined with the right diet promotes weight loss.

- *Improved brain health, memory and cognitive function*—hormonal stimulation as well as oxygen-rich blood help the brain function optimally.

- *Improved skin health*—Your integumentary system is your largest organ and is an organ of elimination. Releasing toxins through the skin from exercise and sweating, can have a profound impact on the overall health of the skin.

- *Pain reduction*—Exercise provides a regulation of all body systems, enhancing the performance of cellular function allowing for the release and regulation of inflammation in the body which causes pain.

- *Sleep regulation*—regular exercise has been proven to aid your ability to sleep well. Physical exertion gives your body the opportunity to burn the energy in your body from all of the food you ate throughout the day. If you do not exercise and continue to consume calories, your body will want to burn the caloric energy in some way, keeping you awake or restless through the night so that the energy can be burned.

- *Improved mood*—Exercise releases serotonin in the brain which is the happy hormone. Your mood will feel more uplifted and happier as a result of exercise.

The one completely overlooked aspect of all the benefits of exercise is that autophagy links to each benefit, causing the outcome to occur. What we feel or see on the outside as increased energy, happier mood, healthier body, and better sleep is the direct result of autophagy.

Every single cell in your body is contacted during the exercise experience. When you look at all of the cells operating as a whole universe of information and regulation, you can see how exercise can benefit not only the muscles and bones but every activity and function of the human body brought out by the action of autophagy. Exercise increases positive stress levels in the body.

The act of engaging the muscles, skeleton, joints, ligaments, and tissues through specific motions causes fatigue in the fibers and even microscopic tearing. Even further in depth, the tears ask for repair through the sophistication of the cellular system, activating and increasing autophagy.

You certainly can create an autophagic response in the cells without exercise; however, for a balanced and healthy experience of healing the body, exercise will always be of benefit to you. Variations on the kinds of exercise and levels of intensity are encouraged and recommended. Overuse of any muscle group or excessive weight lifting can also cause internal damage. It is a fine line to walk, so make sure you know what you are doing before you hurt yourself with exercise. Finding a balance with exercise styles will help improve and regulate autophagy, especially in combination with the other methods for activating this process.

Ch 2.3: Ketosis

Caloric intake in our early days as humans was highly limited. Agriculture wasn't invented yet and people hunted and gathered to survive, covering large distances regularly and fasting between meals. Typical diets were plants, seeds, nuts, fruits, and occasionally meats that were successfully hunted. Animal protein and fat were like drinking at an oasis after a long journey through the desert; it was what the body was ready for after a low calorie to no calorie intake and would replenish the body for more long distances ahead.

Ketosis is the metabolic state where some of the body's energy supply comes from ketones in the blood, rather than a state of glycolysis (glucose in the blood provides the energy). Ketosis will occur when the body is metabolizing fat quickly and converting fatty acids into ketones. It's a nutritional process distinguished by serum concentrations of ketone bodies with normal levels of insulin and blood glucose. Ketogenesis is the formation of ketone bodies that occurs when liver glycogen stores are exhausted, and sometimes from metabolizing MCT or medium chain triglycerides. There are also ketone supplements that you can consume along with your other daily vitamins.

The levels of ketone bodies are regulated mostly by insulin and glucagon. A majority of cells in the body can use both glucose and ketone bodies for fuel. During ketosis, cells can also use free fatty acids and glucose synthesis.

Long-term ketosis can be the result of fasting or keto-diets. Deliberately inducing ketosis serves as a medical intervention for a variety of conditions. During glycolysis, high levels of insulin encourage the storage of body fat and block its release from adipose tissues. In ketosis, fat reserves are readily released and consumed.

There are two sources of ketone bodies: fatty acids in adipose tissue and ketogenic amino acids.

Your adipose tissue can be relied on to store fatty acids which allow for the regulation of temperature and energy in the body. Fatty acids can be released by adipokine, a cell signaling protein, alerting the body to high glucagon and levels of epinephrine, an inverse correspondence to low insulin levels. High glucagon and low insulin relate to times of fasting and also to times when blood glucose levels are low. Fatty acids are metabolized in the mitochondria of the cell in order to produce energy; however, free fatty acids are unable to penetrate cellular membranes due to their negative electrical charge. This leads to an enzyme bond: coenzyme A is bound to the fatty acid to produce acyl-CoA and can now enter the mitochondria.

Now inside the mitochondria, the bound fatty acids are used as fuel in the cells through oxidation, which cuts two carbons off of the acyl-CoA molecule to form a new compound, acetyl-CoA. This new substance enters a citric acid cycle. Citric acid then enters the tricarboxylic acid which creates a very high energy yield in the original fatty acid.

Ketone bodies are also produced in mitochondria and are the response to low blood glucose levels.

During ketogenesis, two acetyl-CoA molecules condense to form acetoacetyl-CoA via thiolase, an enzyme. Acetoacetyl-CoA combines with another acetyl-CoA to form the ketone body acetoacetate. Ketone bodies can be exported from the liver to supply crucial energy to the brain when blood glucose levels are low.

So, what does all of this mean? To break it down simply, ketosis occurs on the cellular level when you are low on glycogen in the body due to a lack of calories or a low carbohydrate diet. Your body burns fat through a sophisticated response and call of the chemicals in your cells. Everything is about balance on the microscopic level.

Ketosis is in balance when the body can burn stored fats. If the body has no fat reserves, or there is no fat being ingested, the body will feed on the proteins or muscles. When your body's insulin is not effectively utilized due to damaged, fatigued and dirty cell waste, ketones can accrue in the body creating a highly acidic internal landscape that can lead to illness and sometimes chronic disease. High acid inside the body is detrimental long term and requires a more balanced pH through the foods you eat, how much water you drink, and your vitamin and mineral intake.

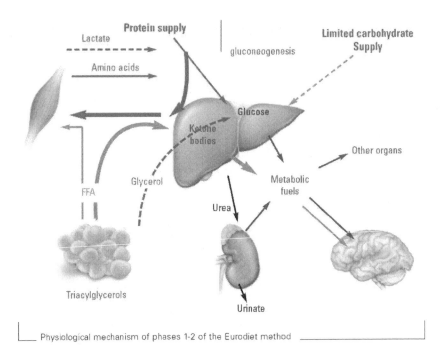

Lactate
Protein supply
Amino acids
gluconeogenesis
Limited carbohydrate Supply
Glucose
Ketone bodies
Other organs
Glycerol
FFA
Metabolic fuels
Urea
Triacylglycerols
Urinate

Physiological mechanism of phases 1-2 of the Eurodiet method

High acid from ketones is known as ketoacidosis and is most often seen in people with diabetes who have issues with insulin regulation. It can also occur in extreme athletes who are overexerting their bodies over long periods with no caloric intake. Think of a triathlete trying to make it to the end of the race after the intensity of the exercises with little to no food. They can also experience ketoacidosis. Another example is childbirth. If a mother is laboring for days without eating, her body can start to react in this way.

Insulin and Ketosis

It is important to understand the role of insulin in ketosis. Insulin is produced in the pancreas, and it is energy, pure energy. Your body's cells use it to regulate proper intake of sugars in the body to operate efficiently. If your cells cannot receive proper doses of insulin, it will be rejected by the cell and end up in the bloodstream. Hyperglycemia is often a result of insulin production that can't release into the cells which chronically occurs and turns into diabetes.

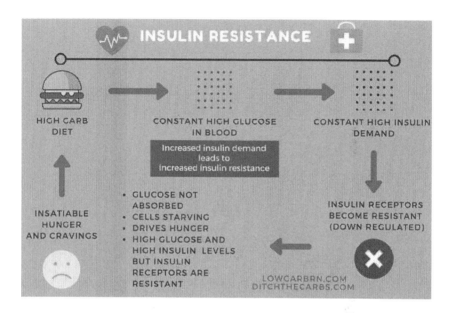

What happens when your insulin production and intake are not effective or functional, is that your energy stores cannot regulate either. And the release of insulin in the blood creates acid or ketones, that lead to an overactive state of ketosis in which you are no longer burning fat. The body holds the fat, keeping you overweight, and starts to lock onto proteins, like the muscle. The exit of ketones from your body occurs through urination, and when you get tested for levels of ketones, it is your body's alert system that you are experiencing functional or dysfunctional insulin uptake due to a chronic overabundance of sugar in the blood. Your body doesn't know how to handle this, so systems begin to malfunction on a deep cellular level.

Here are some important facts you should know regarding insulin:

- Insulin resistance increases your risk of getting diabetes.

- You might be insulin resistant for years and not even know it.

- Insulin resistance usually doesn't trigger any obvious symptoms.

- The American Diabetes Association (ADA) has suggested that up to fifty percent of people with insulin resistance and prediabetes will develop type 2 diabetes if they don't change their diet, exercise, and other lifestyle factors.

- Insulin resistance can increase the risk of obesity or being overweight, high triglycerides, high blood pressure.

- Insulin resistance may develop a skin condition in some people known as acanthosis nigricans. It looks like soft, dark patches sometimes on the back of the neck and armpits.

- A buildup of insulin within skin cells can cause acanthosis nigricans.

You may not be anywhere close to having diabetes; however, insulin resistance over time can lead to prediabetes and eventually type 2 diabetes. Seeing a doctor is the best option, and autophagy can be an added aid in preventing insulin resistance, that leads to diabetes and turning current diabetes around for the better.

Diabetes symptoms:

- Extreme thirst or hunger

- Having hunger, even after having just eaten

- Increased and/or frequent urination

- Tingling sensations in hands or feet

- Excessive fatigue

- Having infections often

There are tests you can take to test your blood sugar levels to find out if you are insulin resistant. The A1C test is the test given by a doctor to help measure your average blood sugar. It may be useful to get tested, so you have an idea of how autophagy can help you become less insulin resistant.

The test measurements look something like this:

- An A1C under 5.7 percent = normal.

- An A1C between 5.7 and 6.4 percent = prediabetes diagnoses.

- An A1C equal to or above 6.5 percent = diabetes diagnoses.

You can also have a fasting blood glucose test which shows your fasting blood sugar level. This test is done after not eating or drinking for at least eight hours.

- Fasting blood sugar levels under 100 milligrams/deciliter (mg/dL) = normal.

- Levels between 100 and 125 mg/dL = prediabetes diagnoses.

- Levels equal to or greater than 126 mg/dL = diabetes.

A glucose tolerance test is another way to diagnose prediabetes or diabetes. Your blood glucose level is determined before this test begins, after which you receive a premeasured sugary drink. Your blood glucose level is then checked again 2 hours later.

- Blood sugar level after two hours of less than 140 mg/dL = normal.

- Result between 140 mg/dL and 199 mg = prediabetes.

- Blood sugar level of 200 mg/dL or higher = diabetes.

According to the American Diabetes Association, if you have insulin resistance, you may prevent diabetes by exercising 30 minutes, 5 days a week and eating a balanced diet. Losing weight can lower your risk of developing diabetes. Imagine what miracles you could work by activating autophagy.

Autophagy is the cleaning crew reaction that begins the change to reorganize cells for better insulin absorption. Without our insulin, the body's sugar levels would derail, and we would only eat off of our tissues. Thankfully, we all have insulin production coming from the pancreas, and can benefit the body by understanding how insulin works and how to regulate our diet and exercise, to allow for proper insulin sensitivity. For autophagy to correct this insulin dysfunction allowing for proper ketogenic performance, a resistance to foods can cause an internal turn of events that allows for proper cell function, namely cell clean-up.

Letting the cells control the dynamic inner world brings about the best body performance. Focusing energy inside the cell, autophagy consumes a great build-up of waste materials that causes the insulin resistance that leads to detrimental disease, and possible ketoacidosis.

What you want from ketosis is a healthy burning of fat fuel. When you are relying on fat stores, you can maintain healthy weight loss and weight consistency. Ketosis is promoted through autophagy, and in order to allow for healthy ketosis, a certain diet must be applied and practiced allowing for fat burning and toxin release.

Complex carbohydrates and sugars are eliminated to renew proper insulin use, performance autophagy, and ketosis. Testing ketosis is a way you can observe if you have activated autophagy in your cells. You can purchase Ketone Strips that change color when applied to urine samples and demonstrate ketone levels in the body, ranging from no ketosis to healthy ketosis to ketoacidosis.

Engaging in the benefits of ketosis will help your body properly produce and utilize insulin, and use fat stores for fuel which assists in healthy weight loss without losing muscle.

Ch 2.4: Fasting

What you don't eat won't kill you, but extensive fasting will starve you to death. There is a fine line to walk regarding fasting to encourage autophagy, and damaging your lifeline connected to food. In reality, no wonder drug can cause an autophagic response in the body. The only way to truly enact the self-eating mechanism of the cell is to deplete the energy in the body by eliminating food.

Your energy is stored in each and every cell inside your system of life. The chemicals produced to create energy in the body release as needed to perform various functions. What if you needed to end the cycle of calories your body receives every day in order to allow for better cell performance?

Fasting gains on autophagy. What this means is that as you reduce the number of calories you ingest in a day you kick start autophagy. While your body is doing less to digest food and circulate nutrients in your body, creating new forms of energy, the cells have a hiatus from exposure to added energy and materials to process and can function to ball up all the garbage and throw it in the recycling bin. It's hard to work in the cell, and most of us aren't thinking microscopically when we eat our daily bread.

Today's diet is extreme. Most Americans eat 3-square meals a day with snacks in between, coffee, sugar, additives, and highly processed foods that are chemically engineered in laboratories, as well as endless quantities of prescription drugs and over the counter medications. On top of all those toxins, the average American is chronically dehydrated, choosing sugary beverages over clean water. There is no way to effectively flush the toxins under those conditions.

What happens when you keep adding calories, limit exercise and refrain from regular water consumption? Disease, obesity, mental and physical stress, mental and physical illness, depression, anxiety, trouble sleeping, inflammation, and more. When you realize the detrimental impact of the American diet on the cellular level, you begin to understand the chronic disease plaguing the nation. The answer is simple: fasting for autophagic performance.

When people think of fasting, they think of rail-thin, bony people who are making a religious or political sacrifice, like Gandhi or the suffragette, Alice Paul. They think of individuals who succumb to extreme dieting methods to lose weight, no matter the cost and end up with psychological disorders like Anorexia Nervosa and Bulimia.

Fasting for health is not starvation. There are limits to consider when approaching this method for activating autophagy. What you find, rather than severe loss of food intake and extreme measures of weight loss, is a carefully regulated and balanced approach to caloric restriction and food elimination. You do not eliminate it permanently; it is a temporary act to elicit the autophagic response.

Many fasts are only 16-18 hours, several days a week, while others may last 24-72 hours with healthy boundaries of when it is too long. Here are a few fasting methods to consider:

- *Time-restricted*—This will include a daily ratio of time that you are not eating and the time that you are. A common ratio is 16:8 whereby you fast for 16 hours and allow food for 8 out of the full 24-hour day. You can adjust the ratio as long as the fasting time is at least 16 hours for a maximum autophagic benefit.

- *Alternate Day Fasting*—Here, you will alternate days you eat with days you don't. Essentially, Monday you eat food; Tuesday you don't. Wednesday you eat food; Thursday you don't, etc.

- *Intermittent Fasting*—This is a full 24+ hour day fast separated by days or weeks. That could look like one day fast once a week or twice a month, or perhaps a 2-3 day fast once a month.

- *5:2 Diet and Fast*—This ratio suggests eating for 5 days and fasting for 2 every week.

- *Low-Calorie Fast*—This kind of fast includes an extreme reduction of calorie intake over a period of time but still allows for some calories to be ingested.

- *Religious or Political Fasting*—This is beyond the scope of this book; however, these kinds of fasts are important to the beliefs of some individuals. It is important that no matter the reason for the fast, you should see to it that you are doing it in a healthy, balanced way.

The basic tactic is to resist food long enough to promote autophagy. Permitting this small fasting time multiple days, a month, or year can reduce your body's cell deterioration significantly.

What you don't want to do, is extend the fast to the point that your body overextends ketosis which causes acidic cell damage, that can lead to fatality and bring about unnecessary starvation,

that causes the body to eat muscle rather than fat stores. This is why engaging in short-lived fasting can provide autophagic cell renewal, while burning fat and restoring optimal cell function.
Dieting has been proven to benefit in the short term; however, most people try to tricking their bodies into losing weight without engaging in autophagy and ketosis. While some diets can be useful under certain conditions and for certain ailments, a majority of mainstream diets lead to insulin resistance, weight retention, and problematic sugar highs and lows that lead to binge eating.

Waste in the cells can easily accumulate under these conditions and without autophagic response initiation, the waste will build, the cells will operate at a dysfunctional or slow level, and balanced health will not be fully restored. Fasting improves the body's ability to restore itself. Taking short breaks from food intake has been scientifically proven to activate autophagy, which allows the cells in your body to clean up and reorganize, leading to a fresher, healthier, more youthful you.

In addition to the overall health benefit of food fasting, research is also showing that autophagy induced by fasting, has an impact on the healing of chronic illness and disease. There have been reports that creating this response in the body while battling cancer, diabetes, and inflammatory diseases can allow for deeper, cellular healing and prevention of future recurrence of the illness that cannot be remedied by prescription drugs, chemotherapy, or surgery.

This is your body intelligence at its finest. We are sophisticated machines that have the capability to self-heal, and creating the autophagic process through careful, healthful fasting could very well save your life.

Ch 2.5: Intermittent Water Fasting

Water is life. No cell in your body can function without it. No living thing on Earth can exist without water's vital essence. Because performance autophagy relates to cell tissue cleansing and renewal, without water, this process would be null and void. The basic human cell is protein, fat, cholesterol, and water. While you begin to increase autophagy through fasting and ketosis, you begin the process of reducing wastes and toxins in the body on a cellular level.

Water will get used to performing all these functions, collecting and disposing of exhausted materials and compounds. The point of energy is to give life to our experience. The point of water is to give life to that energy. Because water is so significant to the system as a whole, water fasting is a described method of autophagy on account of its ability to enhance autophagic reaction and response.

Timing is everything. Intermittence is a level of time which allows your body to receive ample energy through healthy eating and diet, followed by moments and periods of fasting. This alternating effect brings about effective autophagy, giving space and time to the cells to renew and for the body to gain nutrients; both are necessary for optimal health.

Water fasting is the method by which all food is eliminated slowly over the course of several hours and/or days to allow your body time to gently respond and react to fewer calories. Water is then increased to allow for proper autophagic response and activity. The only thing consumed in water fast is water; however, some vitamins and minerals may be consumed for proper internal balance. Although no calories are ingested, some vitamins and minerals are necessary for the proper function of the cells so that they may do their work during autophagy.

Water is essential; it carries all life and acts as the conduit of all internal function and performance. Without it, autophagy wouldn't work. Balancing the fast with extra water is key to healthy autophagic response and brings about greater change, renewal and deep cellular healing.

Chapter 3: Autophagy Performance

The answer to autophagy is in the question of how you want to look at your own health and healing. Too many people are trying to perform at the same level using the same tricks of the trade, flopping back and forth between all of the culturally popular diet crazes, and falling off the wagon on account of highs, lows, and cravings. If you understand how autophagy works, then you also understand that to look at it from the point of view of universal success isn't going to work.

Yes, all of our cells have the same function of cell renewal and autophagy, but no one has the same genetic make-up, DNA, and body type. We can't all fit into the same box, which is why you need to resist the tendency to adopt the program that everyone else is using. We don't have the same reasons for going on diets, exercising, and looking for the cure to health problems. From an outside point of view, it can look the same: weight loss, bigger muscles, long life. However, tapping into the reality of autophagy means truly looking at and listening to your body wisdom.

You are going to heal under the right circumstances for you, but what are those conditions? You can't take the exact same routine from your neighbor and expect the same results; it just doesn't work that way. In order to see a true turn around in your health, you have to tinker with the plan for healing that is unique to you.

Following the instructions of any diet, weight loss, and exercise program can feel like a lot of work. When you fall, of course, there can be a lot of doubt and discouragement that leads to continuing old patterns of eating and digesting. What you get out of autophagy is so much more than the common weight loss program, because it isn't just about weight loss and muscle building; it's about deep cellular healing for long lasting life.

Because our culture stresses all of the weight loss routines and breaking bad habits, we find ourselves pigeon-holed into dieting in short-lived spurts for short term effect, rather than altering the concept of our internal workings and changing our bodies from deep within on the microscopic level. It isn't just how you look on the outside; it's how you feel deep within and how your cells perform and function.

Creating autophagy for health benefits isn't hard. It's not a gimmick or a fad; it's your body intelligence working for you behind the scenes, and all you have to do is create the right conditions for that to occur. You may find some general theories and practices in this book that can help you get started with your renewal program; however, so much of the experience is going to be your own awareness of how your body works and how it doesn't. Your heredity can play a big part in your body structure and body top, meaning that not everyone will look the same when they lose 30 pounds.

Our anatomy is based on the same principles of structure and function that clean and heal us constantly, without obvious notice, but if we are not doing the work to create those circumstances, how can we put that gift to the test? Bringing autophagy to the foreground in your food intake, fasting and exercise cycles can change your whole health and reality.

This chapter will go into greater detail what you can do specifically to enact autophagy through guidelines and steps to understanding each diet, fast and muscle performance so you can fine-tune the healing experience that is right for you.

Ch 3.1: Ketosis Diets

Weight loss occurs for every one differently. We all have our genetic background, healthy or unhealthy eating habits and a long list of favorite snacks and treats that we go, for when we need an exciting pick-me-up. On the day to day level, we pick and graze between meals and have an endless number of options to choose from at the grocery store and restaurants. Many of us enjoy a large quantity of carbohydrates, delicious sugary food and drink, and a hearty helping of premade convenience foods regularly.

All of these factors, from the dietary standpoint, are what lead to the internal cell deficiency that autophagy works to heal. Because we all have our unique internal make-up, it is important to listen to our bodies when beginning to shift into ketosis diets, or keto-diets, as they are often called.

There are side effects of starting ketosis that can cause flu-like feelings that will discourage continuation of the diet. Often times, these symptoms are the result of changing too much, too soon and can be prevented by gently easing into a change in diet, rather than going from zero to 100 mph.

What you can do is slowly start eliminating certain foods one day at a time to control your body's release of toxins. This tactic is known as partial-elimination of these problematic foods. Ranging from days to weeks, careful elimination of these foods will lead to a healthier experience when adopting a new eating plan. Slow adaptation to this new diet will have fewer unpleasant side effects when approached in this way.

Most ketosis diets are relatively similar, but there are a few to consider when looking to create autophagy. They are:

- *Standard Keto Diet (75-20-5)*—This diet involves a ratio of fat to protein to carbohydrates, like the other keto diets will; however, the ratio in this diet usually creates the most noticeable change in the body resulting from fat loss and has a more profound impact overall on activating autophagy. The ratio is 75 percent fat, 20 percent protein, and 5 percent carbohydrates (75-20-5 daily intake). Keep in mind that based on your BMI, or body mass index, the measurements for these amounts will be different from person to person. If you weigh 160 lbs., versus someone who weighs 260, you will need to account for some change in measurement regarding the quantity of food, keeping the overall percentage of daily intake the same.

- *High Protein Keto Diet (60-35-5)*—This diet is similar to the standard keto diet, the only difference being the ratio shift. Rather than consuming 75 percent fat, it drops down to 60 percent, allowing for a higher percentage of protein daily. The reason someone might choose this ratio is if they are working to promote more muscle building rather than fat loss. For some people, starting with the standard diet helps them shave off the fat pounds, and once they have reached that goal they continue the keto diet, shifting to a high protein diet to help build muscle, especially if there isn't a large quantity of fat stores to burn.

- *Cyclical Keto Diet (5:2)*—Like with a 5:2 fasting ratio, this keto diet applies a method for exchanging fats for carbs on a 5 to 2 basis. For the first five days, you will eat a standard ketosis diet. For the following two days, you switch the ratio so that instead of high fat you are eating high carb (70-75% carb, 20-25% protein, 5-10% fat). This diet is often utilized for high-performance athletes who need a major carb load for weightlifting or workouts. It helps to create a balanced fat loss while building muscle mass.

- *Targeted Keto Diet (carbs before exercise)*—This diet is like a hybrid diet of the standard and the cyclical keto diets. You maintain a typical standard keto diet and digest your daily carb allotment half an hour before your workout, allowing for muscle building and stamina in the workout without taking time off of ketosis.

For the best results for autophagy performance, the standard and high protein diets are the best choices for creating ketosis and initiating an autophagic response. The other two diets may be more beneficial on a long-term track and should be considered, especially if you are a bodybuilder or athlete that requires more carb intake for building muscle and using energy.

KETO Food Pyramid

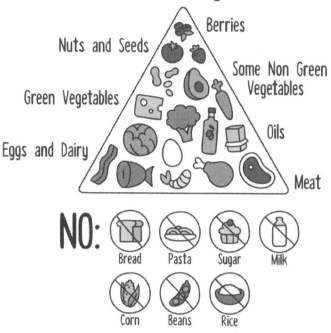

Looking at the standard ketosis diet, you find the ratio of 75 percent fat, 20 percent protein, and 5 percent carbohydrate. Since the diet has almost no carbs, it is essential to start with partial elimination in a week to help avoid those uncomfortable flu-like symptoms. Once you fully eliminate carbs, you can pursue the standard ketosis diet regularly to increase your autophagic performance and overall body health. Some of the foods you will need to avoid eating on the standard ketosis diet are:

- *Sugar*—sweets, candy, juice, soda, energy drinks, sugar additives

- *Grains*—bread, pasta, cereal, rice, etc.

- *Starchy Vegetables*—root vegetables like beets, carrots, parsnips, potatoes, yams

- *Legumes*—Lentils, beans, chickpeas, peas

- *Fruit*—all fruit except small amounts of berries

- *Unhealthy Fats*—canola oil, vegetable oil, margarine, Crisco

- *Some condiments*—condiments that contain any of the above ingredients and especially store-bought mayonnaise

- *Low-Fat food products*—any packaged food that is marketed as being low fat

- *Alcohol*

Foods that you can enjoy on the standard ketosis diet:

- *Meat*—grass-fed beef, pork, poultry

- *Fish*—salmon, cod, tilapia

- *Eggs*

- *Dairy*—butter, cream, some cheeses

- *Nuts* and *seeds*

- *Healthy oils*—olive oil, coconut oil, avocado oil

- *Avocados*

- *Low-Carb Vegetables*—leafy greens, lettuce, peppers, tomatoes, onion, cucumbers, asparagus

- *Herbs and Spices*—salt and pepper and a variety of herbs

The standard diet may seem like it contains very limited ingredients; however, these simple foods can be arranged in countless delicious ways, and there are several delicious recipes specifically for ketosis diets that support this style of eating to support you along the way.

The ratio of foods in the standard diet is that you would have the highest amount of fat, allowing your body to run on fat stores instead of carbohydrates. While burning fat and experiencing ketosis, you ensure a healthy amount of protein so that you don't start eating your muscular protein in the process.

The alternative to that is the high protein version in which you slightly decrease the amount of fat, and increase the amount of protein, leaving the carbohydrate intake the same. The fat ratio goes down to 60 percent with the protein up to 35 percent, leaving the last 5 out of 100 for the carbs. You may elect this method if losing muscle mass is of greater concern, or if you are working on building muscle through ketosis.

The important aspect of why ketosis diets work is that with the high fat-high protein approach, your body will always feel full and satisfied. You will not crave treats, carbs or sugars, especially if you start with partial-elimination of these foods before fully eliminating them from a standard ketosis diet. Many of the diets marketed today don't work because of this issue: cravings. Cravings break the diet and cause a return to the same patterns of insulin resistance and high blood sugar.

It is important that if you choose a ketosis diet for encouraging autophagy performance, you must not eat high fat-high carbohydrate-high sugar. This is the recipe for obesity, diabetes, and countless other diseases of the body.

The necessary program for you is something you will need to tweak along the way, depending on your level of physical activity and your overall goal for health. The ketosis diets are one part of a system that aids in the control of autophagy performance. As you start to incorporate this kind of diet, you can begin adding in intermittent fasts that will continue to offer your body greater opportunity to heal on a cellular level.

Ch 3.2: Steps to Water Fasting

Controlling autophagy can be easy and pleasant with the right approach. After reading about ketosis diets to get you on the right track for autophagy regarding food intake, you can now begin to introduce a greater autophagic response by starting a fast. Plan on giving yourself a couple of months on a new diet before diving into a fast. Allowing time for your body to adjust to anything is healthy. There are some serious key components to consider as well as some precautions and contraindications, before getting started with the steps to water fasting.

When you are considering your water fast, it is important to plan ahead. You don't want to wake up one morning and casually decide that today is the day you aren't going to eat and only drink water (unless you are sick and know that it is necessary). A healthy fast requires preparation and planning and the slow tapering off of food intake.

Figure 1: Intermittent fasting variants

Alternate-Day Fasting
(Eat over 12 hours; fast for 36 hours)

Sun	Mon	Tue	Wed	Thur	Fri	Sat
✖	✔	✖	✔	✖	✔	✖

Eat-Stop-Eat
(Fast or severely restrict calories for 24 hours, once or twice a week or just from time to time)

Sun	Mon	Tue	Wed	Thur	Fri	Sat
✔	✔	✖	✔	✖	✔	✔

Random Meal Skipping
(Randomly skip meals throughout the week)

Sun	Mon	Tue	Wed	Thur	Fri	Sat
B - ✖	B - ✔	B - ✔	B - ✔	B - ✖	B - ✔	B - ✖
L - ✔	L - ✖	L - ✔	L - ✔	L - ✔	L - ✔	L - ✔
D - ✔	D - ✔	D - ✔	D - ✖	D - ✔	D - ✔	D - ✖

Feeding Window
(Eat only during a set period of time every day)

16- or 20-Hour Fast	8- or 4-Hour Eating Window

If you have never fasted, or water fasted before, start with only one day of water only, or try the 16:8 fast. If you are doing a 16:8 fast, you won't need to worry as much about the following steps. Prepare by eliminating meals over the course of 2-3 days prior. Then, you can try one full day of water only. Giving yourself time to eliminate food slowly, before beginning a water fast helps to ensure that you won't suffer issues of fatigue, chronic headaches, nausea, and stomach cramping. Having enough water during a water fast, or any fast, is essential; however, too much water can disrupt your body's balance of sodium and potassium. A range of 10-14 glasses of water through the course of the day is recommended. As you gain comfort with one-day water fasting, you can then begin to allow for longer stretches once or twice a month.

From the one-day water fast, take it up to days and even three if you feel the need, or are prepared to handle that. If you start to feel symptoms of fasting like hunger or dizziness, drink a glass of water and rest. Be gentle with your body. Stand up slowly from sitting or lying positions and avoid strenuous activity and exercise. Meditation and yoga, or gentle stretching will be more appropriate during a water fast.

Attempting to exceed more than 3 days of water fasting may require consultation with a doctor or professional for guidance and aid. Consider what your goals and intentions are before excessive, long-term fasting. Mineral supplements and vitamins may be required for longer term fasts and can even be useful and helpful, in short term fasts. Some of the supplements you can consider using are not limited to the following:

- Sodium

- Potassium

- Magnesium

- Trace minerals

- Whey

- MTC oil (medium chain triglycerides)

- Nutritional yeast

- Collagen

There are some concerns and precautions for water fasting if you have certain medical conditions or diseases. Consult a doctor or professional before fasting if you have or suffer from any of the following:

- Advanced cancer

- Eating disorders

- High doses of prescription medication

- AIDS/HIV

- Alcoholism or drug addiction

- Advanced Type II Diabetes

- Advanced neurodegenerative disorders

If you are pregnant, or post-partum and breastfeeding, avoid water fasting and fasting in general for the health of you and your baby.

When you begin to plan your water fasting, there are some simple steps and guidelines to help you achieve the safest and healthiest autophagy performance. These steps are a good rule of thumb for any fast in general.

Steps and Guidelines for Water Fasting:

1. Plan water fasts when you will not be working and can have relaxing, restful periods.

2. Schedule it so you can first slowly eliminate food before transitioning to water only.

3. Schedule the length of the fast and plan what day you will slowly start to reintroduce food into your system.

4. Have the first foods available on hand before you start your water fast to prevent the need to drive to any grocery stores, in case you are feeling light-headed from the fast.

5. Choose clean, pure water, or distilled water only.

6. Fill containers of water to measure out how much you will need over the length of your fast. Try diving the measured water into to daily required amounts.

7. Reintroduce food with something simple and easy. If you are on a ketosis diet, make a smoothie of leafy greens, berries, and lemon juice, or eat a few spoonsful of high-fat yogurt. Keep it simple and small in quantity.

8. Gradually increase food intake slowly over a few days, avoiding processed foods or overly rich, decadent meals.

9. During the fast, be sure to enjoy lots of rest and relaxation. Do not overexert the body.

10. If feeling hungry, craving food, or having light-headedness, drink 1-2 glasses of water and rest for a while.

Controlling the process of healing on a deep cellular level requires some thought and planning. Engaging autophagy through water fasting can be healthy when approached in a healthy manner. Be sure to ease into a fast, slowly eliminating food, and ease out of it, slowly reintroducing food.

The benefits of water fasting are that you can clean, renew, refresh and restore your body while your internal intelligence cleans, renews, refreshes, and restores on the cellular level.

Ch 3.3: Weight Loss and Water Fasting

Hunger over the course of a water fast is greatly reduced when you start your fast off on the right foot. Energy may start off being lower during the fast, but the consumption of only water from 1-3 days restricts your caloric intake to allow for significant loss in weight. Because of the possible ketosis already occurring from the right diet, your body will already be burning fat stores over muscle allowing for healthy autophagic cell renewal.

What happens then is that during your short-term water fast, you are burning unwanted fat stores and flushing toxins from that stored fat with the water. The result is weight loss.

Loss of weight can get out of hand resulting in your body's instinct to control the loss of fat, hanging onto the reserves for survival. This can lead to taking energy from the protein stores in the body, which is why it is important to balance the fasting with the right diet, right exercise and right rest.

Fasting is believed to be one of the most effective ways to induce autophagy because of the entrance into a state of stress. The stress of this kind relates to the body's ability to engage all systems for survival. When these systems are over-engaged and out of hand, it can lead to severe illness; however, when done properly, recurring periods of timed stress can activate the body's ability to collect and remove waste for the optimal function that allows for survival. This is body intelligence.

Weight loss occurs when you fast, and water fasting actually enhances the ability to flush out what is needing to be released, adding to the overall loss of weight. Effects of fasting, when done properly lead to steady, regulated weight loss.

With the slow transition back to food, you are able to maintain the new weight and experience the rejuvenation on the cellular level caused by autophagy through fasting. There is no current evidence to suggest that weight loss is unhealthy through fasting. When one is properly prepared for a fast, there is less potential for harmful side effects. What you lose in weight, you gain in health.

Weight loss is one of the main reasons people fast. You don't have to water fast only to achieve significant weight loss. You can apply any of the methods of fasting revealed in Ch. 2.4 to promote weight loss; however, the results of water fasting, consuming only water for a period of time, creates a more profound impact on the initiation of autophagy and promotes the flushing of toxins and ketones from the body.

If the goal with water fasting is weight loss in addition to autophagy, be sure to allow time to phase into the right diet. Try incorporating a ketosis diet for 2-4 weeks, or more, before you begin to incorporate fasting. You may already begin to notice significant weight loss from the keto-diet alone. After a period of weeks, or months, you may hit a weight loss plateau and can use water fasting as a kick start to achieving more weight loss. Once you have regulated your diet in this way, you can begin to create a deeper autophagic response by slowly reducing food and calorie intake to enter into a fasting period. Again, you can determine the right fasting method for you by listening to your body, and paying careful attention to what works best for your body type, genetic history, and overall health.

Water fasting is an excellent method for promoting autophagic performance, which leads to healthy loss of weight that you can further maintain and regulate through right diet, exercise and rest.

Ch 3.4: Muscle Mass and Water Fasting

Marketing and advertising show that if you want to bulk up your muscles and keep hard-rock abs, you have to exercise all the time and pack in all the calories you can. Actually, you don't. It is no surprise that if you want to build muscle, you have to exercise, but unless you are a bodybuilder, or weight training for specific sports or athletic purposes, an exercise of various kinds a few times a week is enough to maintain healthy muscles.

Creating healthy eating habits is a must if you want a healthy body overall. If you eat hamburgers every day but go to the gym every day, you may believe that you are effectively utilizing the calories from that fast food meal to build muscle and feel healthy. Reports show that the kind of approach is like a dog chasing its tail. To truly benefit from both exercise and diet to build healthy muscles, a balance is required, as with all things in life.

Autophagy is part of a balance as well. Limiting your food intake for periods of time allows for the pendulum to swing so that your cells have the activity to repair themselves. If we do not create time and space for this, we are out of balance.

Many who consider autophagy as a long-term health plan for a long life and rejuvenation, may find concern about whether muscle mass is lost during fasting periods. This is a legitimate concern, and what water fasting contributes to is the activation of autophagy while resting the body.

During a fast, it is recommended to refrain from excessive exercise or overexertion. Those who have made a habit of exercising every day, may feel like they could lose muscle if they aren't working out at the gym on fasting days. While it would be supportive and healthy to do some light exercise and stretching, there isn't enough evidence to suggest that intermittent fasting can cause muscle loss, even when you aren't exercising. In fact, over exercise, while fasting is what could more likely lead to muscle loss.

The right health plan is entirely up to each person. Only you can know what is working or not working well by listening to your body. Periods of fasting regularly complimented by right diet, exercise, and rest can significantly improve overall muscle performance. When you are not fasting, you can be working on building your muscles through your regular exercise program.

When you are fasting, you can modify your fitness routine to include less weight lifting and cardio, and more stretching, gentle resistance and deep breathing work. You can simply go for a walk around the neighborhood to engage your muscle groups while in a fasting period. Not all exercise needs to be powerlifting and cardio to support healthy muscular build.

With fasting, less is more, and balance is essential. There won't be a loss of muscle when water fasting; there will be activation of autophagic performance which leads to the prevention of many diseases, illnesses, and health disorders, and there will be a gain of optimal cellular function, rejuvenation of cells, and regulation of hormones and body systems.

Ch 3.5: Extended Water Fasting

Beyond the general promotion of autophagy through the right diet, exercise, fasting, and rest, there can be uses and reasons for extended fasting. Extended fasting may be something that lasts as little as 4-5 days or as much as weeks. Planning an extended fast means you probably have a good reason for it.

It could be regarded as a deeper healing measure for more chronic toxic release or disease reduction. It could also be intended for religious or political purposes that are based on personal beliefs, faith, and values. Other than that, for health, there are not a lot of reasons to explore extended water fasting. If you choose this method of autophagic performance, you will need to consult a medical professional or nutritionist who can provide some guidance and support.

There can be great dangers to the system as a whole with extended water fasting and seeking advice on mineral and vitamin supplements, and a scheduled plan for eliminating and reintroducing food is necessary for the healthiest benefit. Three to five days is doable when you want to cleanse, detox, and initiate autophagy. When you begin to exceed a week, you will need to have an appropriate support and plan in place.

The best method for prolonged or life-long autophagic performance is through intermittent fasting coupled with the right diet, exercise, and rest. Very sporadic, extended fasting may be useful for certain reasons, but consultation with a doctor or professional is advised for the healthiest experience.

Chapter 4: Optimizing Autophagy

The right diet, exercise, fasting, and rest are something you will know when you lock onto your need for autophagy. This need could alter over time, or it may be that you don't need every aspect of it in the same way for the rest of your life. All of the research on autophagy has shown that you don't need to do it every day, but you may find times in the course of your life that you will need or want to activate it on a daily basis. You may lose all the weight you set for your goal, using all four components, but will need to adjust your approach to autophagy once that goal is reached.

Life is long and changes daily. There will never be any diet, form of exercise, or fasting ritual that has to stay the same forever unless you are practicing these experiences for religious purposes. We grow, we transform, we change, for our whole lives and so should the food we eat, the kind of exercise we get, how often we fast, and what kind of rest is best under the circumstances.

We don't have the perfect relationship with these factors in a perfect way on all days of the year; we will ebb and flow and need to understand our responsibility to ourselves to pay attention, especially if you want to use autophagy regularly to enhance your health and renewal.

Significant research on the overall impact of prolonged autophagy has not been known yet; however, many improvements are being seen and experienced in the overall health of those who include performance autophagy activation in their regular health plans. You can guide yourself along the way using the ideas laid out in these chapters to help you determine the focus of your needs for inducing autophagy.

Bringing into focus all of the components of chapter 3, this chapter will outline the best methods for optimizing autophagy for deep cellular healing. Let your cells do the dirty work while you plan the routine, and handle the steps and instructions for initiating an autophagic response. Allow for some room to grow and shift. You don't have to follow these guidelines to a T; you can experiment and explore different ways of doing it that work best for your personal, optimal health.

Renewal is easy when you bring the right ingredients to the table. This chapter will give you the steps you need to change your diet, exercise, fasting routine, and resting time, in order to fully enhance autophagy. The four categories together promote the ideal healing platform. Remember, the recipe is in your hands, and you have the power to heal.

Ch 4.1: Right Diet

Taking what you know about how autophagy works and how to activate it, you can begin with the first important steps to creating that internal response. The next steps will give you the approach you need to shift and transition into the right diet. The right diet will initially be a keto-diet for the best autophagic response and weight loss, depending on your goals. A modified diet down the road will be beneficial as well; keeping your body healthy means listening and responding to its needs. A long-term keto diet can be adjusted to allow for more carbohydrates.

To begin a ketosis meal plan, you need to ease into it, like you would ease into a period of fasting. The reason for this is that when you immediately stop eating all the foods you are used to eating, such as bread, pasta, sugar, fruit, and many other items, you can enter a shock phase. For some, it can feel like illness, and there can be headaches, cravings, and fatigue. It can feel a lot like the flu. Your body has been eating certain foods for a while, and to suddenly deprive the body of these things can create an inflammatory response.

To create a smoother transition from your current eating habits to a keto-diet, you will need to break it down into phases and allow for some time. Week 1 will be the first phase of transition, eliminating some of the foods that you need to avoid to create ketosis. Week 2 will be the second phase of further elimination and increase in fat and protein. Here is a breakdown of what that may look like:

Phase 1: Elimination

- Alcohol

- Unhealthy fats like canola oil, vegetable oil, mayo, margarine, imitation butter

- All processed, low-fat foods

- Condiments containing sugars and carbs

- Most grains, including pasta, cereal, bread. You can keep small quantities of grains during phase 1, like rice, quinoa, and barley.

During this elimination, you are taking away some significant carbohydrates but are still allowed to eat some carbs and sugars found in fruit, starchy vegetables, legumes, and other sugary foods and beverages which will prevent a significant body shock. A possible weekly diet for Phase 1 could look like this:

Monday

>*Breakfast*: eggs and bacon with tomato and mushrooms
>*Lunch*: Salad with salmon and fruit on the side
>*Dinner*: Chicken soup with rice

Tuesday

>*Breakfast*: yogurt and berries with a tsp of honey and 3 tbsp of almond slivers
>*Lunch*: BLT on whole grain bread
>*Dinner*: Steak and potatoes with broccoli

Wednesday

>*Breakfast*: Fruit bowl with yogurt

Lunch: Salad with chicken and quinoa
Dinner: 3 bean soup with sausage and veggies

Thursday

Breakfast: Goat cheese and basil omelet with tomatoes
Lunch: Salmon and asparagus cooked in butter and lemon
Dinner: Roast chicken with carrots and potatoes

Friday

Breakfast: Poached eggs with tomatoes and kale
Lunch: Codfish with steamed vegetables and butter
Dinner: Beef Stew

Saturday

Breakfast: Fruit and nuts
Lunch: Turkey lettuce wraps
Dinner: Roasted pork shoulder with vegetables

Sunday
Breakfast: Eggs and bacon with a spinach feta salad
Lunch: Salad niçoise
Dinner: Baked Salmon and broccoli

This weekly diet starts to prepare you for an even bigger elimination of carbs and sugars, increasing fat and protein.

Cooking with healthy fats like olive oil, coconut oil, and avocado oil is encouraged in Phase 1 and should be adhered to in Phase 2. You can also cook with a small amount of butter or clarified butter known as ghee.

There are many keto-diet cookbooks that contain specific cooking recipes to help you avoid incorporating any foods that you are working to eliminate. Avoidance of alcohol during phase one is important. Your body converts alcohol into sugar, so it is like drinking glasses or pints of candy. Increase water consumption and try more herbal teas. One of the reported side effects of ketosis is bad-breath. This is caused by ketones being released in the body from burning fat and can be evident in your breath. Rather than chewing sugary gum or sucking on sweet mints or lozenges, try a few cups of peppermint tea between meals. Adding freshly squeezed lemon juice to your glasses of water is a wonderful digestive aid and can help with balancing internal pH levels. You can also use apple cider vinegar in place of lemon juice to create the same effect.

Stay away from processed, packaged foods and try to prepare meals with fresh ingredients for the best results. Let go off all the protein and power bars, all the cookies and snacks, all the pastries and flavored lattes. Let go of all the bread and baked goods, all the food made with canola oil and corn syrup. This is what you begin to do in Phase 1. Give this phase some time. It doesn't have to be only one week. It may feel more comfortable for you to extend this phase into 2 weeks or more while your body adjusts. And be sure to drink plenty of water throughout.

Phase 2: Elimination

- All grains including any remaining bread, rice, quinoa, etc.

- All fruit, except small portions of berries

- All sugars and sugar additives, including honey and any beverage containing sugar

- Legumes—beans, chickpeas, etc.

- Starchy vegetables like beets, carrots, potatoes, yams and parsnips

During this elimination, you are further letting go of any remaining carbs and sugars. The standard ketosis diet allows for 5% daily intake of carbs in ratio to your fat and protein consumption. You can get these carbs from berries and some quantities of vegetables.

In Phase 2, you will be incorporating more of the high fat/high protein foods your body needs to stave off hunger and cravings, allowing your body to enter enhanced stages of weight loss and ketosis. A typical weekly diet with full elimination could look like this:

Monday

> *Breakfast*: spinach and goat cheese omelet with three eggs
> *Lunch*: tuna salad with feta, olive oil, and lots of leafy lettuce greens
> *Dinner*: pork chops with kale salad and broccoli

Tuesday

> *Breakfast*: yogurt and berries
> *Lunch*: big green salad with one avocado, cucumber, celery, green bell pepper, cabbage, toasted walnuts, and an olive oil lemon dressing
> *Dinner*: salmon and asparagus with butter and lemon

Wednesday

Breakfast: bacon and eggs with tomato and basil, side salad
Lunch: guacamole with celery and cucumber sticks, a handful of nuts
Dinner: pesto chicken and roasted broccoli and brussels sprouts

Thursday

Breakfast: mushroom, spinach, tomato-basil omelet
Lunch: chicken salad lettuce wraps
Dinner: steak and eggs with salad

Friday

Breakfast: poached eggs on an arugula salad with feta and olive oil
Lunch: roasted pork loin and steamed veggies
Dinner: tilapia cooked in butter with sautéed broccoli, kale, and spinach

Saturday

Breakfast: yogurt and berries
Lunch: toasted nuts, one avocado, smoked salmon and celery sticks
Dinner: roasted turkey breast with a side salad

Sunday

Breakfast: omelet with scallions, mushrooms, cheddar
Lunch: salad niçoise

Dinner: roast chicken and brussels sprouts

Keep in mind that while cooking for a ketosis diet, if you need snacks between meals, eat nuts and seeds, or another kind of protein snack. Use healthy oils and clean ingredients. Do not use canned vegetables.

The Phase 2 diet has removed sugars, most carbs and increased proteins and healthy fats. Use ketosis recipes and cookbooks to help you adjust measurements based on your own weight and BMI. Additionally, if you are going to enjoy breakfast or snack items like yogurt and berries, be sure that you are choosing full-fat yogurt that does not contain any added sugars or flavorings.

Finding the right supplements for you can also improve the quality of your daily nutrient intake. Many herbal teas are packed with minerals, vitamins, and nutrients. Having a hot cup of tea between meals can stave off hunger, while soothing and warming the belly, helping it to feel full while packing in minerals and antioxidants.

Bone broth can be an excellent supplement to some meals as it is very filling and nutrient dense. Broths can also be useful in phasing out food to begin transitioning into a fasting period. Bone broths are simple and easy to make at home. You can purchase some quality bone broths from the store, but if you are cooking chicken for your ketosis diet, you can freeze the bones until you are ready to make broth and then put them in a crockpot overnight with purified water. Add some onion and celery for flavor. There are several recipes available for broths, and you can use a variety of bones, not just chicken.

Broths are soothing to the intestinal lining, providing a healthy space for nutrient absorption. Adding bone broths into your daily meals can be a huge improvement to your quality of digestion. You can have a cup of broth instead of tea or skip breakfast or dinner and just enjoy a cup of hot broth.

Finding ways to enjoy the program your body is undertaking can feel like a challenge at first, but initiating the process is part of the pleasure of starting your journey to healing. A cup of broth or a handful of your favorite nuts can go a long way.

Every person is different, weighs a different amount, and has a different health history. Finding the right recipes for you will help you feel like you can satisfy and satiate your hunger.

Ketosis diets are in full, popular swing, and there are numerous delicious recipes to keep you on the right track. Engaging in a ketosis diet while enjoying some of the other autophagic activation methods will ensure a whole healing, whole body process.

Ch 4.2: Right Exercise

Get yourself ready to move your muscles. There isn't a time in your life when exercise will have no value or benefit. It is always a good idea to include exercise in your life. The limits of exercise depend on the person and the goals being worked toward; however, whatever exercise is chosen, you will add to the output of autophagy.

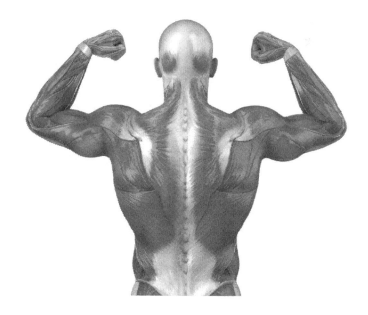

When you dial into the kind of exercise that works for your frame, build, performance goals, and intentions, you can expand on that exercise in various ways, creating the right routine for you. The key is finding something you enjoy. You don't have to program yourself to exercise like everyone else. In fact, that can cause burn out and avoidance. The right exercise is what is right for you.

Most exercise routines or plans promote some level of variety.

This is essential to a balanced, physical health plan. What you choose depends on you, but within your routine, there should be a balance between resistance training or weights, cardio, balance, and stretching.

For optimal autophagy performance, there needs to be a flow within each of the methods. Doing the same exercise routine 6 days a week is not going to benefit anyone, long-term. Different muscle groups need time to recover and heal after the stress and strain of healthy exercise.

Here are some examples of some possible weekly workouts to promote autophagy:

Example 1:
Monday: Calisthenic Routine
Tuesday: Yoga
Wednesday: Weights
Thursday: Rest
Friday: Calisthenic Routine
Saturday: Yoga
Sunday: Walking with weights

Example 2:
Monday: Stretching for one hour
Tuesday: Barre/Pilates class
Wednesday: Rest and water fast
Thursday: Power walking with weights
Friday: Swimming Laps
Saturday: Rest and water fast
Sunday: Pilates

Example 3:
Monday: Weight lifting
Tuesday: Jogging for an hour
Wednesday: Rest and 18 hours fast
Thursday: Stretching and walking with weights
Friday: Swimming
Saturday: Rest and water fast
Sunday: Yoga

There are numerous ways you can plan an exercise routine, and if you begin to feel bored with it, you can change it! You may want to have a gym membership so that you have access to the equipment, machines and swimming pool, or you may prefer a home work out set up so you can easily exercise whenever you need to. You can acquire weight sets, stretch bands, yoga mats, and medicine balls to have available for use at any time. A little a day goes a long way.

Calisthenics

A majority of people today are aware of things like yoga, running, weight lifting, and all the different types of fat burning cardio workout you can find. Many people, though, are not as familiar with calisthenics. They are common enough exercises, but you may not have heard the name before. If you have heard of Cross Fit, then you understand calisthenics.

It is essentially a series of regular motor movements like standing squatting, walking, running, swinging, etc. that uses your own body weight for resistance and strength building. You really don't need a lot of machinery or equipment to use this kind of exercise. Many gyms offer training like this, providing a variety of different movements in a routine so that your whole body gets a full work out. You can also find several online videos that can guide you through a full calisthenic routine, many of which do not require any equipment.

Whatever method or schedule of exercise you choose, the right exercise is what is right for you, and all exercise will benefit your overall health, wellness, vitality and most importantly, autophagy.

Ch 4.3: Right Fasting

Not all the answers to health and wellness or weight loss and muscle health come from just diet and exercise. The connection that autophagy has to overall wellness and optimal body function, has been proven through research and studies over the past several years. A great number of autophagic performance results come from the practice of periodic fasting.

What can benefit you most during fasting is the planning and organizing of how and when you will fast for autophagic activation. There are several approaches to fasting and all of them can be useful at different times for different purposes. The ones that will be most effective for autophagy in combination with the right diet, exercise, and rest will allow for periods of time with no food at all and water consumption throughout.

These periods can last as little as 16 hours or as long as three days. A common fasting practice is the 16:8 ratio. What this means is that you eat nothing for 16 hours and eat 2-3 meals within 8 hours. That could look something like this:

- 7 am—wake up and drink water and tea

- 12 pm—eat

- 3 pm—eat

- 7-8 pm eat

- 8 pm-12 pm the next day FAST

This is what daily fasting looks like, and depending on your hunger levels, you may only need two meals and a snack or just 1-2 meals. That is something you have to gauge on the day of the fast. This works well because your body is naturally in a fasting state when you sleep. When you wake up, instead of having breakfast right away, you wait until lunchtime to have your first meal and then have until 8 pm to satisfy your hunger. After 8 pm, you can drink water and herbal tea but will avoid food or snack, as well as alcohol. You can repeat this daily for continued benefit.

Another method of fasting that permits longer autophagic response is a longer fast, supported by healthy eating and transition on either side of the fast. An example of this type of fast can look like this:

Monday: skip breakfast, eat lunch and dinner

Tuesday: skip breakfast and lunch, eat dinner

Wednesday: very light dinner only

Thursday: water fast

Friday: water fast

Saturday: drink hot tea in the morning, broth midday, a small amount of yogurt

Sunday: broth in the morning, light lunch, light dinner

Monday: breakfast, lunch, and dinner

You can extend the length of the water fast to cover more days, or you can water fast for only one day out of the week, depending on your goals and intentions. You may find as you become familiar with the fasting experience that it is easy to shift back to food, without too much discomfort.

Another type of fast involves regular eating five days a week followed by 2 days of very light eating. You may not experience the most optimal autophagic response, but it will be activated by the extreme calorie reduction over the course of the 2 days.

When you decide how you want to fast, the right experience for you will be one that can occur at times where you can rest and not work, especially if you are water fasting. Incorporating the right diet and right exercise over the course of a week can look something like this:

Monday

> *Breakfast*: skip breakfast, *Pilates with weights*
> *Lunch*: tuna salad with feta, olive oil and lots of leafy lettuce greens
> *Dinner*: pork chops with kale salad and broccoli

Tuesday

> *Breakfast*: skip breakfast, *yoga*
> *Lunch*: skip lunch, water with lemon, and a cup of broth
> *Dinner*: salmon and asparagus with butter and lemon

Wednesday

> *Breakfast*: skip breakfast, water with lemon, *one-hour stretching*
> *Lunch*: skip lunch, herbal tea
> *Dinner*: salad (drink water throughout the day)

Thursday

Water Fast: water throughout the day, *resting, meditation*

Friday

Breakfast: skip breakfast, hot tea and *yin yoga*
Lunch: hot broth, small salad with light dressing
Dinner: steamed vegetables with butter

Saturday

Breakfast: omelet with tomato and basil, *cardio workout*
Lunch: toasted nuts, one avocado, smoked salmon, and celery sticks
Dinner: roasted turkey breast with a side salad

Sunday

Breakfast: omelet with scallions, mushrooms, cheddar
Lunch: salad niçoise, *Calisthenics*
Dinner: roast chicken and brussels sprouts

You can repeat this fasting schedule every week and just play around with the recipes and exercise you do, or you can alternate weeks that you are fasting and do a 2-3 day fast twice a month.

The right fast for you is something to explore. Working to create optimal autophagy means allowing for periods of zero calorie intake, not just when you are asleep, so you can enjoy the maximum benefit of deep cellular healing. Find the fast that is right for your body. You may need to do some experimenting to make sure you can incorporate intermittent fasting into your lifestyle, diet, exercise, and rest.

Ch 4.4: Right Resting

Part of healing is allowing periods of time for your body to regenerate. Autophagy is a powerful, internal intelligence. Your body has the power to heal itself, but if you are not offering it the proper time to rest, you will be digging a deeper hole to clean up later.

Starting off on the right foot and creating good, healthy habits for wellness is essential to locking down the results you are looking for. In our current culture, everything is fast-paced, instantly gratified, and we are all plugged in all day long to our devices. Many people have 40-60 work weeks that make it challenging to find time for rest, let alone diet, exercise, and healthy fasting.

Bringing your health into focus includes allowing for proper periods of rest. During your experience in activating autophagy, it will be important to organize time for your body to rest. Rest is important after significant exercise. When you strain and stress your body, it requires time to recover and repair microscopic damage to the muscle fibers and tissues.

When you eat a meal that is filling, it is helpful to enjoy a period of rest after to allow your body the proper amount of time to digest. Your body can focus on digestion better if you offer it the rest to do so.

Fasting is something that can temporarily lower your energy since you are not ingesting any calories. It is common to experience some fatigue under these circumstances. It is a great opportunity to incorporate rest for your body while it is fasting. Imagine too, on the microscopic level, when you are resting your body is undergoing great healing, transformation and change, performing autophagic response from the intermittent fasting.

Many people consume large amounts of sugar and caffeine daily to bump them out of slumps that occur throughout the day, after meals, after long periods of work, or because of lack of sleep the night before. If you replace your caffeine and sugar doses with moments or periods of rest throughout the day, you would aid your body in a much healthier way, eliminating the need for caffeine and sugar altogether.

Sugar is the antithesis of a healthy diet and optimal autophagic performance and should be avoided anyway if you are planning on activating autophagy. Caffeine is regularly consumed by most people, and it is not discouraged in the majority of diets. The longer-term effects of daily caffeine intake can be as detrimental to your body as any other stimulant or toxin. Successful autophagic performance doesn't need caffeine and like other foods and beverages that hinder health. It should be avoided and replaced with herbal teas, water, and other non-caffeinated beverages.

You can ultimately rest better without it, and if you are getting the rest you need, you won't need caffeine at all.

The right rest comes with experimentation, awareness of your needs, listening to your body, and responding to it when it is asking for rest. Incorporating the right rest will fluctuate depending on day to day life, activities, exercise, diet, schedule, and more.

Rest is vital to supporting optimal autophagic performance. All four components together bring about a level of health, that will deliver clear results that you can see and feel. Activating autophagy through the combination of right diet, exercise, fasting, and rest is the key to a long and healthy life.

Chapter 5: Autophagy for Everyone

There is no one alive who doesn't have the internal intelligence to heal themselves. Creating a domino effect for autophagy to support a long and healthy life through the use of a certain diet, exercise and fasting is a choice you can make if you are ready. Activating this process is normal and is part of the inherent work of the basic human cell.

No matter where you are on your journey toward healing and healthy living, learning how to activate autophagy brings about a process of deep, cellular healing that renews and rejuvenates all the cells in your body preventing various diseases like diabetes, cardiovascular disease, neurodegenerative disease, and more. Other impacts involve the balance of hormones, healthier skin and hair, reduced inflammation, increased metabolism, stronger immunity, and revitalized cellular functions that allows for enhanced function in all body systems.

Transformation of the whole body occurs when you learn to activate the natural cleansing process all the way down to your cells. The focus of this book is to offer the reader information, understanding and steps to help begin this process on your own. There are many studies and reports, testimonials and evidence to offer further details about the benefits of autophagy. This chapter will cover some of these topics, including frequently asked questions, myths, and endorsements from people's personal success with autophagy performance and health.

Ch 5.1: Frequently Asked Questions (Regarding Autophagy, Ketosis, and Fasting)

Question: What is autophagy?

Answer: Autophagy is a process on the cellular level by which cytoplasmic material such as dead organelles, oxidized proteins, and other scraps are transported to the lysosome in the cell for recycling.

Question: Why is autophagy beneficial?

Answer: It is a key process in a healthy functioning human body and is key to preventing diseases such as liver disease, various forms of cancer, neurodegenerative disease, autoimmune disease, and acute or chronic infection, to name a few. It also has a variety of anti-aging benefits because of the way it refreshes cells.

Question: Why do ketogenic diets promote autophagy?

Answer: Ketosis diets drastically reduce the intake of carbs to almost nothing and increase fat intake significantly which creates a drastic shift in energy, from glucose to ketones. This energy transition acts similarly to a fasting state, thereby leading to an increase in autophagic performance.

Question: How long does it take for autophagy to activate?

Answer: When glycogen is expended or drained through fasting, autophagy is activated, usually after 12-16 hours.

Question: If on a keto diet, how often should you intermittently fast?

Answer: Studies suggest that limiting long fasts to a few times a year can be beneficial, but that short 16-18-hour daily or weekly fasts are acceptable on a more regular basis and create more profound autophagy. It varies from person to person.

Question: Is fasting dangerous?

Answer: Fasting for 1-3 days is usually not a problem for healthy individuals. If you are not already on or working toward eating, a healthy diet, or if you have a chronic disease, such as liver, kidney, or heart disease, you may be at risk. Consulting a doctor before fasting is suggested if you are not sure if you are in a healthy state for it.

Question: How much weight loss can be expected with fasting?

Answer: It depends on many factors, such as how many calories you already eat a day, if you exercise and how long you are fasting. If you eat 2,000 calories a day, you may end up losing around 2-3 pounds on a 3-day fast. Losing more than that in a week could mean a loss of muscle rather than fat which is why healthy fasting is so important.

Question: How much will I lose with ketosis?

Answer: It depends on many factors, such as current weight and health, exercise, etc. On average, once your body starts ketosis, you may lose 1-6 pounds in the first week. After that, weight loss slows down to 1-2 pounds a week. If you are on a long-term ketosis diet, you will gradually lose weight more slowly. If you hit a plateau, it may be a good time to shake up your diet and branch out before returning to a standard ketosis diet.

Question: How do you increase autophagy?

Answer: Exercise. Fasting. Low carb diet.

Question: How often should I attempt intermittent fasts?

Answer: There are several methods, and you will have to find the one that feels right for you at the right time. Methods include 16 hours fasting/8 hours eating every day; % days regular diet/2 days fasting or restricted calorie intake; 24-hour fast 1-2 times a week; every other day fasting; fast all day and eat one big meal at night.

Ch 5.2: Myths About Autophagy

Myth: Fasting-induced autophagy causes starvation in the body.

Answer: Fasting is not starvation; it is taking a break from eating.

Myth: Autophagy eats away at your muscles when you fast.

Answer: Your body has ample resources in the form of glycogen and fat all over your body. If you are intermittently fasting, the first thing your body will do is go for the sugary glycogen, then the delicious fat before even considering the protein of muscle.

Myth: You will be malnourished if you fast to increase autophagy.

Answer: Fasting does not equal malnourishment, and as long as there aren't calories involved, minerals and vitamins are permitted if there is a concern of losing nutrients. Malnourishment is not attainable in a short-term fast unless you have a pre-existing medical condition.

Myth: The most important meal of the day is breakfast.

Answer: This slogan is propaganda from a time long gone. Scientific studies, advances in technology and research, and the experiences of many individuals have proven that is ok to skip breakfast.

Myth: Intermittent fasting is not good for your health.

Answer: Studies show that periodic fasting has numerous health benefits all of which relate to the activation of autophagy caused by fasting.

Myth: Keto diets are too high in fat and are bad for your heart.

Answer: Studies and research indicate that it isn't fat and cholesterol that cause heart problems; it is high carbohydrate, low-fat diets that create an unhealthy dynamic that leads to cardiovascular issues. Having high or low fat, high carb, and high sugar is the worse combination.

Myth: Keto diets allow you to eat all the butter, bacon, and steak that you want.

Answer: While ketosis diets are high in fat and protein, depending on your height, weight, and body mass index, it is important to regulate the amount of each based on your unique body profile. It won't be the same for everyone and unlimited bacon is not for everyone either.

Myth: Keto diets are the best way for anyone to lose weight.

Answer: No diet is perfect for everyone. Keto diets may not be right for you. All bodies are different, and so it is important to listen to your body to determine if keto diets are the best choice for you.

Myth: Fasting will cause hunger and overeating.

Answer: It isn't always a lack of food that causes hunger and overeating; it's eating too much all the time. Your body will always be expecting more sustenance on schedule, especially if you are always eating 3-square meals a day plus snacks in between. A lot of foods available are full of additives, preservatives, and sugar which you become addicted to and crave. Removing foods like this from the diet will dampen cravings and overeating. Fasting will create energy, vitality, and clarity.

Myth: Keto diets are a long-term solution.

Answer: While utilizing ketosis diets for weight loss and to promote autophagy can be beneficial, eventually you may need to find a more balanced solution. Your body will eventually need carbohydrates again for optimum health. Using keto diets periodically after a major weight loss, alternating with other healthy diet plans may be the best plan for long-term health.

Ch 5.3: Testimonials

"I have been overweight my whole life. Since I was a child, I ate food for comfort and was always heavy. I tried diets but ended up gaining weight in the process. A friend told me about her weight loss with ketosis diets and how it helps your cell regenerate in your body. The first few weeks, I lost 16 pounds with exercise and intermittent water fasting. I had never tried fasting or ketosis before and wasn't sure what to expect. It has been a year, and I have lost 38 pounds and feel wonderful. I still use water fasting periodically to help maintain my weight. I have so much energy, my skin is glowing, and I have more self-confidence about my health than I ever have in my life."
-Jeanine, 35
California

"I started bodybuilding in college going to the gym multiple times a week, eating a high carb, high protein diet to pack on the muscle. After a few years, I still wasn't at the level of weight training and muscle density that I wanted. Sometimes, I would feel a little sluggish before and after workouts. I saw a YouTube video about autophagy and how it can improve your health by cleaning the cells throughout the body. With the fitness programs and diet I was on, I learned that I needed to take it to the next level in my health outlook. I switched to a ketosis diet that allowed for some extra fat loss I needed which helped define my muscles. I started periodic water fasting and did carb intake on work out days only. The improvement in my muscles and energy was phenomenal, but I also felt great from the inside. No more sluggishness. It was like a light switch turned on, or my body got flushed and cleaned."
-Chad, 29
New York

"I tried a number of prescription drugs to help with my arthritis. They all seemed to work ok until I stopped taking them. I didn't like the side effects of taking them. I was never the sort of taking medication and have been healthy most of my life. I started looking for alternatives and discovered fasting with water only. I read several stories of people who were able to turn their inflammation around and live pain-free. I started with a trial fast to see how it felt, fasting and resting one day out of the week. I also cut out a lot of sugar, caffeine, and alcohol that were causing flare-ups in my arthritis. After a month of water fasting one day a week, I was able to stop taking the arthritis medication. I continue the fasts twice a month and have gotten rid of inflammatory foods and drinks from my diet. Now I can go on those long walks along the beach I enjoy so much."
Phillip, 63
Florida

"When I found out I had chronic fatigue syndrome, I was relieved to know what I had been struggling with in my health for the past few years. The downside was that none of the doctors seemed to have a cure for the symptoms. I started to do research online to see if any other people with chronic fatigue syndrome had had any success with medications or other methods. That's when I heard about autophagy. I began to change my diet and to exercise with a moderate routine three days a week. I started noticing a change right away when I tried a keto-diet, but it wasn't until I started fasting once a month that I really started to feel a big difference. It took several months of fine tuning my diet, exercise routine and when to fast, but now, a year and a half later, it is almost as if I cured myself of chronic fatigue."
Darcy, 42
Missouri

Conclusion

You are a living organism full of potential. You have everything you need within you to promote a healthy life. Changing your diet, exercise plan, and other factors is one thing; doing it to activate a deep, internal healing process is quite another. When you begin to look at the root cause of all the obesity, illness, stress, and short-lived lives, you can see that it is not just about what fitness and health magazines are promoting. You have to understand how your body is working hard to heal you from within.

In this book, you learned the basics of autophagy, what it is, and how it can literally change your health. You have also been given precautions, guidelines, and steps to activate autophagy in your own cells. It is happening on some level already, but you have the power to kick it into high gear to get the healing results you are looking for. You can renew, rejuvenate, and refresh your whole body with a few key components: right diet, right exercise, right fasting, and right rest.

Now that you have the knowledge of how to begin activating autophagy in your body, you can start making changes to help promote and support this process regularly. Try a few different ways and approaches and see what works best for your body. The right approach is just right for you. There is no diet or exercise program that is universally perfect, but autophagy is a part of us all. Start from there and watch your health transform. Finally, if you found this book helpful or useful in any way, a review on Amazon is appreciated. Enjoy!

Image Bibliography

Human cell
http://www.slideplayer.com/slide/3858464

Lysosome
http://www.studyread/importance-of-lysosomes

Healthy vs Unhealthy Cells
http://dreamlifecrew.wordpress.com/2012/06/13/you-need-tre-en-en/unhealthy-cell

Autophagosome
http://nature.com/articles/ncb1007-1102

Types of Autophagy
http://novusbio.com/research-areas/autophagy

Ketosis
http://sites.bu.edu/ombs/2013/10/15/ketosis/

Insulin Resistance
http://adventistvegetariandiabetics.wordpress.com/diabetes-basics/articles-about-insulin-insulin-resistance

Keto Food Pyramid
http://universityhealthnews.com/daily/nutrition/keto-diet-health-benefits-of-ketogenic-diet/

Fast Schedule
http://examine.com/nutrition/the-low-down-on-intermittent-fasting/

Muscles
http://sciencedrivennutrition.com/caloric-restriction-and-your-muscles/

Intermittent Fasting for Women:

Learn How You Can Use This Science to Support Your Hormones, Lose Weight, Enjoy Your Food, and Live a Healthy Life Without Suffering from Your Dietary Habits

by Serena Baker

Introduction

Thank you so much for downloading *Intermittent Fasting for Women*. Congratulations are also in order because you've just accepted taking on one of the biggest missions towards health that you could imagine. You're about to embark on a journey with intermittent fasting to see what healing you can accomplish for your mind, body, and soul. And you'll be surprised to know that the potential for healing is great.

Stop right now if you're not female-bodied. This book is about the specific effects of intermittent fasting on specifically *female* neurological, cardiovascular, digestive, regenerative, etc. health over time. If you're on female hormones for whatever reason, you'll likely find this book helpful; if you're a woman in any regard, you're definitely reading the right book.

The following chapters will introduce intermittent fasting to female readers through both scientific fact and personal advice. My name is Serena Baker, and I'm interested in helping you through this introduction to intermittent fasting because I'm passionate about your ability to heal yourself through an altered pattern of eating.

I'm a single mother, so I don't have time to mess around with foods and lifestyles that don't provide constant, quality nutrition to my kids and myself. I've always been passionate about healing myself through the right foods and exercise, but as you'll come to read, intermittent fasting just made a lot of things "click."

These days, I've recently received my bachelor's degree in Nutrition, and I make it my work to share this information about health, fitness, and nutrition with as many women as possible. Intermittent fasting is my focus in particular, but as a single mother, it's always been other women on whom I center my sharing of knowledge with.

When I first learned about intermittent fasting, it was before I had my degree, and I didn't even realize I was doing it. I was just doing what felt right for my body, eating within eight hours each day and waiting about four hours after waking up to eat. I thought I was just more conscious of when I felt hungry, but it turns out I was actually practicing intermittent fasting without knowing it.

When I picked up a fitness book and read about intermittent fasting, I was absolutely intrigued. A lot of the effects listed had been happening to me, and the logic made so much sense. It appeared intermittent fasting was encoded in our genes to be beneficial because our ancestors might not have been able to eat constantly. Those hunters/gatherers would have had to intermittently fast much longer and more often than we did, and yet they survived!

They more than survived — they thrived! And then I read that our bodies and brains got kick-starts from the physiological effects of IF. Everything made sense. Finally, I came across a section on the 16:8 method of IF. I realized that the lifestyle I'd chosen for health was a well-established nutritional choice. When I used to eat three full meals each day and have the occasional snack, from morning to evening, I'd feel so foggy, groggy, and irritable. After I intuitively switched to the 16:8 method of IF, I became more conscious, present, healthy, and able to work like I was able to in the past.

What started out as a health-based choice for me became a lifestyle adjustment immediately because the effects were just so valuable in my life that I couldn't just do it a day or two each week. With sustained effort, I became able to lose that persnickety extra twenty pounds that had been hanging around, and I felt more energetic than ever. More than just my weight, my energy level was affected, too!

My doctor commented on how my blood pressure had reached healthier levels, and as an asthmatic, my breathing got better once the weight was off and the blood pressure went down. It was a glorious time, and it all happened to be backed by the science of nutrition. Of course, I went on to study nutrition then, to figure out how to help others, so that's how we've come to this moment.

In the following pages, you'll learn about what to do, what method to choose, what to avoid, and what happens if you're stressed, breastfeeding, working with PCOS or autophagy, or menopausal. At the end of this book, 12 recipes will be provided for your work with weight loss and IF.

I hope that you learn a lot from this book and feel empowered to try IF for yourself! I also wanted to say that there are a good number of books like this one on the market, but I promise you, you're in good hands! Let's go on and get started!

Chapter 1: Intermittent Fasting for Men vs. Women

As a book oriented towards women, we have first to establish how and why the female body works differently from the male body, as well as what specifically needs to be adjusted for IF women versus IF men. Female and male anatomy involves different hormones, different bodily arrangements, and different neurological connections. And with different bodies come different responsibilities.

When it comes down to it, females' abilities to carry their children within their bodies means that the body can very easily tell when the individual is starving, and it won't allow that person to have children at that time. For women, this message is more urgently felt than for men, and that uniqueness for the female body will be described fully in this chapter.

In the following pages, we will begin by describing the sciences of sex difference and nutrition, and then we will explore how these two things interact through a discussion about male vs. female bodies' reactions to hunger. Next, we'll establish (and remind of) several reasons why sex distinction when working with IF is productive, and we'll end this chapter by going over a few points to tie everything together.

By the end of this chapter, you should feel knowledgeable, validated, inspired, and ready to consider undertaking IF shortly. You should understand how IF will affect you because you're female, and you will likely still have a lot of questions about the procedure ahead of you. That curiosity is totally valid, and all your questions will be answered in time. To start, let's look at the science of the human body.

The Science of the Human Body

Have you ever wondered why it happens to be that you eat more when you're hungry than you're hungry for? Have you ever been curious about why you sometimes can't stop even when you know you're full? As someone coming to IF with goals of weight loss, you likely are very familiar with these frustrating feelings, but if you're coming to IF with goals other than weight loss, you might not be as familiar.

Regardless of your experience with hunger and whether or not you're able to stop eating when you feel you're full, there are scientific reasons why the saying "Your eyes were bigger than your stomach!" exists. First on this list of reasons is the existence of hormones leptin and ghrelin. Both leptin and ghrelin seem to have a large effect on regulating appetite, and subsequently controlling fat storage and gain.

While leptin is secreted from fat cells in the stomach, heart, skeletal muscle, and placenta in females, ghrelin is secreted basically only from the lining of the stomach. Despite where the hormones come from, however, they both end up affecting the brain. Leptin decreases feelings of hunger, while ghrelin does the opposite. Leptin and ghrelin both end up communicating with the hypothalamus in the brain about stopping or starting to eat, but their effects are divergent.

Insulin is another hormone that our bodies produce that effects our health in several ways. For instance, insulin is produced in the pancreas, and it helps regulate the amount of glucose in our blood, but if someone's insulin levels are too high or too low, his or her weight is imminently affected. With low insulin levels, one can't help but lose weight, but too low of insulin levels can be dangerous because the body needs sugar to use as energy. The trick is finding a healthy balance while working to lose weight.

If you're overweight or working with IF, your hormones' signals to the brain become affected. If you're obese, for instance, the signals are interrupted and distorted, while for those working with IF, those signals are triggered not to go off as frequently through an altered pattern of eating.

One final element to note in this section would be the thyroid, whose function is essential in determining both health and ability with weight loss. The thyroid regulates hormones that affect the speed of your metabolism, and if your thyroid is over- or under-worked, your health, energy level, and weight will certainly be affected. In order to lose weight, you'll want to speed up your metabolism without hurting or overworking your thyroid, and that can be tricky to work out properly sometimes.

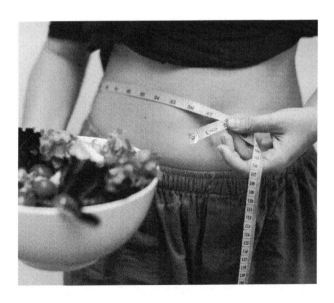

How the Male vs. Female Bodies React to Hunger

When it comes to the science of the human body, everything matters, from the foods we eat to how often we eat, what hormones we allow to produce, which ones we limit, and how well our thyroids are working.

When you're hungry, your body sends signals to the vagus nerve in your brain, and it communicates a lot of details. It reveals how empty (or full) your stomach happens to be, the nutrients that are processed in the intestines, and what deficiencies may be present in the body as a whole. After the stomach sits empty, it starts to grumble (a process called "borborygmus," which pushes any remaining food into the intestines to be digested fully), and then your stomach and intestinal walls begin producing that hormone, ghrelin, that makes you feel hungry.

If you're female and you tell yourself you're not hungry when you get this feeling, your brain often doesn't work in your favor. The hypothalamus and vagus nerve get triggered, making you feel hungry even if you keep telling yourself you can't eat yet or aren't mentally hungry. In the male body, however, the physical hunger sensations and hormone secretions can be limited in effect to the brain through inhibitive thoughts against hunger and eating.

Furthermore, a study on female versus male rats from 2013 revealed that when females (opposed to males) fast for a few days at a time, their abilities to control that hunger response become more fine-tuned than males' do, leading to their ability to lose more weight overall than the male rats could. This study clearly applies to humans' experiences with intermittent fasting as well.

Reasons for Sex Distinction with IF

The primary reason why there is a separation of males and females in the study regarding IF is that the reproductive organs of males and females are different, making their responses to intermittent fasting dissimilar. With different reproductive organs and different reproductive capacities, these two sexes will have different sets of hormones being produced at different times and being sent to very diverse spaces in the body.

Ultimately, it is true that these two sexes will have different responses to fasting about weight loss potential and reproductive health. As the rat study from 2013 reminds us, females can lose weight faster through IF than males can, but they also have restricted abilities to have children during those times of IF (while males don't), which absolutely reaffirms the importance of sex distinction in studies of (and practice with) intermittent fasting in the human world. Different bodies respond differently to things that jolt the system like IF, and it's truer to say that each's process with IF will be dissimilar. However, the first step is making distinctions based on sex and hormonal realities so that the individual comes out of the fast as healthy and energetic as possible.

When it comes down to it, noting sex differences about weight loss work with fasting helps refine the process of IF for the individual. With these differences taken into account and planned for, the results of the fasting lifestyle change are better, meaning more productive, less restricting, and more beneficial for the health of the individual overall.

Points to Consider

While we'll get into this section with more detail later, it is important to note that there are certain experiences, character traits, and body types that are less productive for someone who wants to lose weight through intermittent fasting. Sometimes, you're better off growing as a person first, while other times, you're better off *gaining* weight rather than losing it, even if you can't see that yet.

Additionally, intermittent fasting is not an end-all or an all-cure for health and weight loss. Especially for those individuals who are listed in chapter 4 later on, if you feel like you still need to lose weight when your doctor suggests otherwise, you might be better off working through your issues with a trained and licensed psychologist or therapist before you put an IF plan into action.

Finally, it may go without saying but just to express it now, if you're ever feeling dangerously light-headed or low-energy, or if you lose your period while you're working with intermittent fasting, go to a doctor as soon as possible. Discuss how to move forward as safely as you can or switch your eating back to a more standard pattern or timing so that you can reset and start again with better forethought and planning.

Chapter 2: Intermittent Fasting as a Woman

Because it's so important to divide research and studies of IF between men and women, I wanted to make this book oriented towards only women's health and productivity with weight loss during times of intermittent fasting. That being said, there will be no more mention of men in this book. We'll focus on women and get straight to the point.

When you engage with IF as a woman, you will encounter struggles unique to your body. You may have to tweak your method, your timing, and your approach numerous times until you perfect your practice to what's the most healthy and productive for you. This chapter will go over some of the basics of your hormones, your body, and your mental health, all about what IF can do for the situation inside.

By the end of this chapter, you should be armed with information that will strengthen your IF practice and help you know how to succeed even when you come up against internal hardship. You should feel more confident in how to alter your eating pattern to kick-start your metabolism without losing any of the good things your body does for you. You should feel interested in beginning or planning your lifelong intermittent fast.

Hormones & Health: Weight Loss

When it comes to female hormones, reproductive health takes internal and unspoken precedence over the weight concerns of the conscious individual. This primacy of reproductive health stands out more so with females than it does with males, as we discovered in the last chapter through the 2013 rat studies and more. However, there have to be bigger biological reasons behind that increased sensitivity.

The cause seems to be kisspeptin, which is a molecule similar to a protein that helps neurons communicate with each other about hunger and energy and more. This molecule exists in both males and females, but females have far more kisspeptin than males do, making them even more sensitive to energetic changes in their internal balances.

Therefore, when females' bodies release hormones like leptin, ghrelin, and insulin (that make them feel hungry or full), their brains and internal systems are already that much more inclined to "hear" those feelings and respond to reestablish balance. Women are therefore more likely to struggle with weight loss and general health problems related to increased sensitivity. Despite your body's natural processes, however, you can *absolutely* learn how to make intermittent fasting work for you and still maintain your ideal weight, health, and productivity.

IF & the Female Body

Since intermittent fasting is not so much a diet as it is an altered pattern in eating times and frequency, its relationship with the female body is not the same as the standard diet's relationship would be. In fact, it's not necessarily supportive for females to practice a strict diet while intermittent fasting, for the combination of the two, can work serious havoc on the female body itself.

To counteract any curious side-effects of IF on your physical and mental states, you can try and make sure to eat as nutritious a selection of food as you can, whenever possible. Furthermore, you can try not to *over*exert yourself through exercise, especially since you're altering your food and nutrition intake significantly. Also, you can ensure that you're not forcing yourself to engage in IF if you're ill, suffering from an infection, or struggling with a chronic disorder of some kind. Finally, if your body is already exhausted from work or struggles with anxiety (or otherwise), you might not want to put yourself through additional stress with a new pattern of eating.

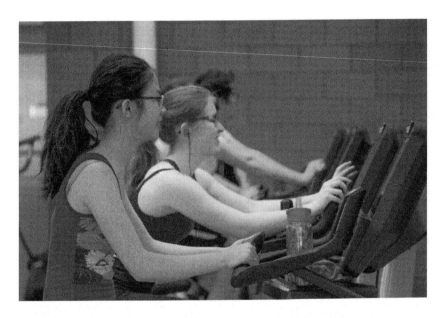

The most important thing to do as you begin to engage with intermittent fasting as a female-bodied person is to make sure you're as connected to (and introspective of) your body as you can be, as often as you're able to be. The more you know your body and its tendencies (i.e. the frequency of your period, your tendencies with metabolism, your fat storage areas, your most common moods, your emotional crutches, etc.), the more successful your experiences with intermittent fasting can be.

Physical Effects of IF for Women

While the general effects of intermittent fasting include increased energy overall, clearer cognition and memory, improved immunity, slowed aging process, better heart health, increased insulin sensitivity, and more, are some of the physical effects for women deserve a little more detail in specific. For women, those specific details include:
lowered blood pressure in about two months or less, lowered cholesterol by ¼ the original toxic amount, better blood sugar control, decreased likelihood for type 2 diabetes, lowered chances of cancer, potential for increased muscle mass (with the ability to preserve it longer!), increased lifespan by up to 50 years, and increased awareness of internal bodily processes in general.

After a few months of intermittent fasting practice, you're sure to feel that your senses are somewhat heightened compared to how they were before, that your body works better and smoother than ever, that your weight melts off like wax from a candle, and that your mind and cognition are clearer than ever before.

Some physical effects function almost like warning signs for the woman practicing IF, too. If you experience poorer skin conditions, complete insomnia, loss of hair, excessive or shocking decrease in muscle mass, loss of period entirely, heart arrhythmia, or increased inflammations (whether internally or externally), you'll definitely want to consider altering your process, stopping the IF for a while, or visiting a nearby doctor for advice.

Using IF to Help with Periods, Fertility, and Metabolism

If you struggle monthly through painful periods; if you know you don't want to have children and you're not concerned about future fertility; or if you want to kick-start your metabolism to help yourself lose weight, all you have to do is start intermittently fasting without any concern whatsoever. If you're looking for hard and fast changes for your harsh menses, your fertility, or your weight issues, work your way up to fasting a few days a week, and you're sure to see the side-effects you seek played out within a month or two.

If you're interested in getting help with painful periods without substantial effects on your future fertility, simply make sure to get enough fat in your diet and supplemental estrogen (which you can find over the counter in a variety of forms). By making sure to consume enough healthy fat and by not restricting your caloric intake too much, you can use intermittent fasting to ease difficult menses without it having too much effect on your metabolism at the moment, and with it having hardly any effect on your fertility later on.

If you want the metabolism boost without effect on your periods or fertility, here's what you can do. Make sure you're eating enough healthy fats, but restrict caloric intake slightly, not too much though, mind you! You don't want to hurt those hunger hormones or inhibit your ability to ovulate and have a healthy period!

For these reasons, you should make sure *not* to intentionally or fastidiously "diet" while you're intermittently fasting but seeing as how you *do* want to lose weight and kick-start that metabolism, you can do *something* to help your body remember not to hang onto too much excess! That *"something"* that works so well is two-part: (1) once you define your method, keep to its timing strictly and; (2) when you have your meals, don't overindulge, binge, or gorge yourself; allow your caloric intake to be limited, but only slightly, as you work with IF.

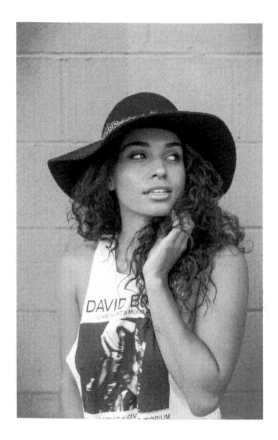

Chapter 3: Diet & Intermittent Fasting

Because you'll likely want to keep your reproductive and menstrual systems working to their best capacities while you engage in intermittent fasting, you'll have to make sure your dietary choices reflect the health you want to see. You won't really want to "diet" all that much, as mentioned above, but you can make certain healthful changes that allow your body to function at its highest capacity *while* it adjusts to intermittent fasting, sheds that excess weight, and reaches a new and purer energy level than you've ever experienced before.

In this chapter, you will be introduced to concepts and details that will help you eat and drink the things that are best suited to your overall growth and success with intermittent fasting. You'll be shown the pros and cons of the intermittent fasting lifestyle, and you'll be taught tips on how to manage hunger and generally achieve your IF goals.

By the end of this section, you should know the best and worst that intermittent fasting has to offer, and you should feel confident that the foods you'll seek during your break from fast will be as health-conscious and supportive as possible, based on the information you've gained. Finally, you should also feel prepared to deal with those "worsts" that IF has to offer through the tips at the end of the chapter. If you're not ready to try intermittent fasting by the end of this section, I'll be incredibly surprised.

Pros & Cons of IF as a Dietary/Lifestyle Choice

On the most basic level (without being too redundant), the pros of switching to intermittent fasting (whether as a lifestyle choice or as more of a simple two-month fasting experiment) include:

- Increased health overall
    - through weight loss, lowered insulin & blood sugar levels, heart health, better muscle mass preservation, increased neuroplasticity, potential for cancer healing, lower blood pressure & cholesterol, healthier hormone production, longer life, re-started/re-inspired nutrient absorption, reduced inflammation

- Increased energy, improved mental processing and better access to memory

- Increased overall sense of well-being
    - both mentally and as a side-effect of having the body type you want through weight loss

- Eased & regulated menstruation
    - including lessened period cramps and potential for lessened fertility

- The ability to retain your current diet and caloric intake

- The overall simplicity and ease of starting and maintaining your IF approach, and the versatility and flexibility of IF as a practice

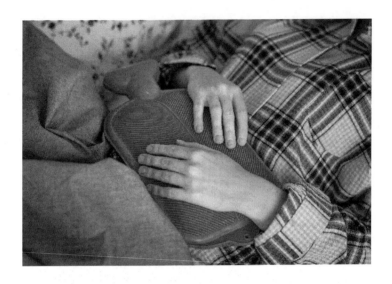

On the flip-side, the cons associated with intermittent fasting (as both a lifestyle and momentary dietary choice) include:

- Potential for increased headaches
  - These are often caused by dehydration and salt withdrawal from eating less than normal.
  - Increase your water intake & mix in a quarter-teaspoon of salt with each water glass, and you'll feel right as rain in no time.

- Potential for constipation
  - Just increase your fiber intake to help with this issue!

- Potential for dizziness when in a fasting period
  - Look to the final section of this chapter for help in this case.

- Potential for muscle cramps

- Take supplemental magnesium or sit for a while in an Epsom salt bath to cure these "growing" pains.

- Potential for worst-case-scenario side-effects
  - This potential is only a concern if IF is not practiced the right way for you and your body.
  - potential side-effects include: irregular or ceased menses, hair loss, dry skin/acne, slow healing to injuries, mood swings, super-slow metabolism, constant cold feelings, insomnia, etc.

- Potential to binge when you do eat
  - Be conscious of your body and what it can handle!

- Interference with social eating patterns
  - It might feel awkward not to eat with everyone else, or to have to explain yourself every time you don't.

- Low energy or unproductivity during fast periods
  - This issue can be helped with practice and by eating the right types of foods when you do eat.

- The fact that some of the lasting effects of IF are still largely unstudied or uncertain
  - such as: its effects on the heart, on fertility, on breastfeeding women, on stress, etc.

What Foods & Liquids Do

When you go about your first round of intermittent fasting, you'll need to know what to avoid and what to keep close at hand. The following portion of this chapter will reveal exactly what's safe, what to avoid, and what does what for you.

When it comes to foods, the best things to have around are:

- All Legumes and Beans – good carbs can help lower body weight without planned calorie restriction

- Anything high in protein – helpful in keeping your energy levels up in your efforts as a whole, even when you're in a period of fasting

- Anything with the herbs cayenne pepper, psyllium, or dried/crushed dandelion – they'll contribute to weight loss without sacrificing calories or effort

- Avocado – a high-, good-calorie fruit that has a lot of healthy fats

- Berries – often high in antioxidants and vitamin C as well as flavonoids for weight loss

- Cruciferous Vegetables – broccoli, cauliflower, brussel sprouts, and more are incredibly high in fiber, which you'll definitely want to keep constipation at bay with IF

- Eggs – high in protein and great for building muscle during IF periods

- Nuts & Grains – sources of healthy fats and essential fiber

- Potatoes – when prepared in healthy ways, they satiate hunger well and help with weight loss

- Wild-Caught Fish – high in healthy fats while providing protein and vitamin D for your brain

When it comes to liquids, some of it is pretty self-explanatory:

- Water:
  - It's always good for you! It will help keep you hydrated, it will provide relief with headaches or lightheadedness or fatigue, and it clears out your system in the initial detox period.
  - Try adding a squeeze of lemon, some cucumber or strawberry slices, or a couple of sprigs of mint, lavender, or basil to give your water some flavor if you're not enthused with the taste of it plain.

- If you need something other than water to drink, you can always seek out:
  - Probiotic drinks like kefir or kombucha
    - You can even look for probiotic foods such as sauerkraut, kimchi, miso, pickles, yogurt, tempeh, and more!
    - Probiotics work amazingly well at healing your gut especially in times of intense transition, as with the start of intermittent fasting.
  - Black coffee
    - Sweeteners and milk aren't productive for your fasting and weight loss goals.
    - Try black coffee whenever possible, in moderation.

o   Heated or chilled vegetable or bone broths
o   Teas of any kind
o   Apple cider vinegar shots
    ▪   Instead, try water or other drinks with ACV mixed in.

Drinks to avoid would be:

- Regular soda

- Diet soda

- Alcohol of any kind

- High-sugar coconut and almond drinks
  o   i.e. coconut water, coconut milk, almond milk, etc.
  o   Go for the low-sugar or unsweetened milk alternative if it's available.

- Anything with artificial sweetener
  o   Artificial sweetener will shock your insulin levels into imbalance with your blood sugar later on.

Managing Hunger & Other Useful Tips

A few supportive tips to help troubleshoot, keep inspired and stay focused as you may happen to encounter the "cons" of intermittent fasting are as follows.

Generally, keep these pointers in mind: don't over-exercise and over-limit yourself with calorie intake or with food when you do breakfast. Take pictures of your progress to help keep the inspiration flowing, try not to binge when you breakfast and make sure to do your proper research or check with your doctor to be sure your plan for intermittent fasting is really the right one for you!

When it comes to managing hunger, the best thing to do is think of hunger like a wave passing over you. Sometimes the build-up to that wave seems unbearable, but it will crest and crash eventually, passing completely over and through you. If you wait it out, keep yourself busy, and take a few sips of a drink instead. You'll find that these hunger pangs are bearable and not quite as overwhelming as they were at the start. By the end of the third day, you should have a significantly increased capacity to handle these feelings of hunger.

If you start feeling dizzy or lightheaded, one of two things is likely happening to you. You may be experiencing low blood volume, or you might be experiencing low blood *pressure* instead. Just drinking water, in this case, might not help you all that much; in fact, if you just drink water, you'll be diluting the number of electrolytes in your system even more, so try mixing a bit of sea salt in your water instead. Frequently, for those who don't experience dizziness or lightheadedness unless they're intermittently fasting, this addition of sea salt to water does the trick. However, some people were liable to feel dizzy or lightheaded before they ever tried IF. For those people (or for those for whom mixing salt into their water doesn't help), taking magnesium supplements can also work well, and if that still doesn't help, the issue could be something else entirely. Possible adrenal weakness, anemia, or low blood sugar would most likely be the cause in this case.

If your period gets lighter or starts to disappear, make sure you're getting enough fat in your diet when you fast! If you *had* been limiting calorie intake, stop doing that right now, and be sure not to binge (on the opposite extreme). Just eat what you would if you weren't IF or dieting at all. These slight adjustments should help resolve this issue. If not, seek advice from your doctor.

When you notice you've become moodier, there are a couple of things you can do to help and troubleshoot the issue. First things first, don't open yourself up to negative moods by keeping the information about your eating pattern shift to yourself and people you really trust. Some people will bombard you with questions, hate, or confusion when you tell them about your work with IF, and you should remember that you *don't* have to tell anyone who you think won't support you.

Second, you can make sure you're not still in the detox period of intermittent fasting! During the first few weeks, you'll be working through the detox period that brings up lots of literal stink and emotional issues to boot. Bear through the trial period and see if that moodiness lingers. If you're still frustratingly and unusually moody after week two is complete, you might just have low blood sugar. Work to counteract low blood sugar through the foods you choose to eat when you breakfast, and the issue should clear itself up in no time.

Finally, two pieces of advice are left, and they're some of the most important ones to internalize. First, choose a plan that starts small and incorporates your life in its planning! If you sleep for almost 12 hours each night anyway, the 16:8 method might be best for you. If you wake early without much sleep constantly, you might be better off doing alternate-day fasting. Go with what works for your schedule, and things will start off so much smoother than they would otherwise.

Second and lastly, start with one month and be open; see what happens! You're bound to get frustrated and moody after and during the first week but commit to withstand the awkwardness and at least get through the first two weeks to the beginning of week three. Stick with it and wait to see what this unintentional cleanse has in store for you.

Chapter 4: When to Avoid Intermittent Fasting as a Woman

While intermittent fasting is flexible, versatile, and adaptable to many different lifestyles, it is still the case that many women should probably *not* attempt IF, for the sake of their overall health. Chapters 7, 8, 9, & 10 will go on to discuss four additional types of women that should be especially cautious proceeding with intermittent fasting, but still, for these women, things *can* be productive when practiced the correct way. Conversely, there are a handful of types of women that aren't well-suited to intermittent fasting in any fashion, for the sake of their lives or others, and this chapter is dedicated to these women.

The following pages will address five different profiles of candidates who wouldn't be conducive to growing and healing with the intermittent fasting meal plan. Of course, the sex distinction in our studies of intermittent fasting plays a huge role in this chapter, for the intersections of sex and disease or disorder are what makes these candidates so problematic about IF itself. From the pregnant candidate to the underweight woman, the female patient with the eating disorder, the female diabetic, and the woman with the troubling personality, it remains true that intermittent fasting isn't necessarily for everyone.

However, even with these limitations in place, there is lingering potential for each of these types of women to come to a place of progress or healing eventually that would allow them to move through their struggles and attempt IF at their own pace. Therefore, if you qualify as any of the following candidates, don't be too dejected or hopeless! With the appropriate personal growth and the right lessons being presented to you, you'll surely come back to intermittent fasting as soon as you're ready for it.

Exploring the Pregnant Candidate

Although intermittent fasting can give you increased energy, better metabolism, and stronger cellular protection, the risks clearly outweigh the benefits for pregnant IF candidates. Since the female body is made to bear children, the effects of intermittent fasting are already debated in their relation to female health, but when it comes to pregnant and soon-to-be mothers, the answer to the question is a clear "No." Pregnant women should not be working with intermittent fasting.

For the expecting mother, long periods between meals are not necessarily such a good thing. The pregnant woman will need to be eating whenever she's hungry to gain the weight and nutrients her future child will need to survive. Furthermore, she will need to combat the morning sickness and nausea that go along with pregnancy, and if she's concerned about her timing with the intermittent fast, she might put herself in a detrimental situation for her overall health by mistake.

If you're recently pregnant but had used intermittent fasting previously with great success, you can shift back to focusing on *what* you eat rather than *when* you eat. Just as it is for the standard person shifting from normal eating to intermittent fasting and going from *what*'s eaten to *when* it's eaten, when you switch from IF to pregnancy, you'll shift eating habits once again. This time, however, you'll try to make sure you're eating the best foods whenever possible; not just in your okayed eating windows.

If you're having trouble stopping your intermittent fast while you've just become pregnant, you might want to reconsider the reasons behind your IF in the first place. Is it really for your health, or does it support your controlling tendency to limit your weight? Try to make sure that when you're pregnant, you're looking for what supports your health, rather than your mental image of what you should look like and what you think you should weigh. Pregnancy is a beautiful time, but it's not about restriction, it's about abundance and weight gain and growth, so it doesn't mesh well with IF at all.

Exploring the Underweight Candidate

For women who are already underweight, intermittent fasting might not be the best thing for your health. Surely, there are unintentionally underweight women who don't have the time they'd like to have for eating or who don't have the energy they'd like to have for cooking, but there are also intentionally underweight women who are looking for an additional method to use to keep off that "excess" weight for good.

If you're incredibly underweight already (even if you don't feel like it!), steer clear of intermittent fasting. If you're only five to ten pounds underweight and you're seeking spiritual enlightenment, lessened brain fog, or a jolt to your digestive system, IF may work just fine for you without being problematic. (While you *might* find a method of IF that works alright for you in this case, don't make the hard and fast decisions on eating pattern switching without first making sure to consult a doctor or health professional.)

Essentially, the problem arises when the individual is already over 10 pounds underweight, for these individuals aren't giving their digestive systems a break or a free moment for healing by switching to IF. Instead, the individual in this stance forces his or her digestive system to claw at itself and scrape at the bottom of the barrel to try and heal itself. I shouldn't have to explain why that simply *won't work*.

Overall, something you can use to determine whether you're in the healthy or unhealthy weight range is your BMI (Body Mass Index). If your BMI is anywhere between 18.5 and 25, you're in the healthy weight range. However, if you're lower than 18.5, be cautious about attempting intermittent fasting. If you're lower than 17, definitely do *not* try this method, for your body can't stand to lose anything else, and to choose IF would cause extreme detriment to your health rather than aid it.

Exploring the Candidate with an Eating Disorder

For the individual with an eating disorder, no matter what variety, intermittent fasting may seem to be helpful, but it will only function as a trigger for that person's disorder. No matter who you are, if you approach intermittent fasting for healing or weight loss, you're probably doing so because you want to switch from stuffing yourself of emptiness to healing yourself with goodness. Your focus, in other words, likely falls on growth (not physically but emotionally, spiritually, mentally, and regarding health capacity) rather than withering.

For the individual suffering from an eating disorder, all attempts toward health and growth are skewed by distortions of body image and self-esteem. Essentially, all attempts toward health and growth are twisted by the compulsory drive to purge. If you or someone you know struggled or struggles with anorexia, bulimia, orthorexia, binge eating, purging, avoidant/restrictive food intake disorder, or any other eating disorder, be extremely curious and demanding with them if they share an interest in intermittent fasting.

Question their inspirations and drives; demand they are honest with you. The likelihood is greater than not that this person is using intermittent fasting as a way to lose weight they can't afford to lose rather than to get healthier in general. If you're able to discern it at all, the individual's reason for *starting* IF is the best way to ascertain their true intentions. It can be hard to tell who has an eating disorder and who doesn't, but the way people talk about food, body image, fasting, and dieting can reveal more than you could ever anticipate. And once you *can* tell who has an eating disorder, help them stay clear from IF because it can really exacerbate their circumstances despite their (and your) best intentions.

Exploring the Diabetic Candidate

If you're already on insulin, as a diabetic most likely, you're already working to keep your levels of blood sugar at balance. If you add into the mix IF work to increase or decrease insulin resistance (to help with weight loss), you'll put yourself in a truly dangerous spot. People with diabetes should absolutely *not* skip doses of insulin to lose weight by lowering blood sugar. This would be disastrous for someone who has diabetes because they'd surely lose the weight, but they'd feel drained to a disastrous degree because humans do *need* this sugar or glucose in our blood to derive energy.

So, if you have diabetes, stay away from intermittent fasting. It's unfortunate, I know, but this type of eating pattern change will do absolutely nothing good for you. As with the pregnant candidate, you could try to switch the foods you're eating instead of when you're eating. By adding the right, healthful foods into your diet, you might find that the weight that sticks to you so stubbornly can be depleted with your condition being made none the worse. However, be careful if you're diabetic when it comes to *fasting disguised as dieting*. If you feel inclined to try a juice or liquid diet, second guess those inclinations, for it's very likely that this type of diet would cause extra stress to your system, what with the high glycemic and fiber-free contents of some juices.

Basically, if you're diabetic and feeling inclined to make your life healthier, don't limit *when* you eat and don't just drink liquids. Rather than restricting whatsoever, try to *incorporate* healthier, more whole foods that are oriented towards healing innately and then maybe add exercise into the mix when you're ready for it.

Exploring Problematic Character Traits

While the previous entries in this chapter have to deal with physical traits and conditions, this final one has to do more so with personality and character attributes instead. The truth of the matter is that some personality types will not mesh well with the lifestyle connected to intermittent fasting. Whether you're controlling, OCD, impatient, moody, reserved, or just too young, you're not in for a "treat" by taking the first steps toward the intermittent fasting lifestyle. Nevertheless, the fact holds that if you can work through your struggles and face your (personality) demons, you might find yourself changed by intermittent fasting in ways no one would have ever expected.

Controlling people expect the world to be easily manipulated to suit their needs, urges, and comforts. Unfortunately, the world doesn't often act so easily shapeable, which puts controlling individuals in tough places. In fasting and dieting especially, control goes out the window and natural progress/timelines take its place. Therefore, controlling individuals might have trouble adjusting to intermittent fasting. Although these people will be able to make changes to their techniques as they go along, they still won't be able to actualize the changes they want with any immediacy. For controlling people, working with intermittent fasting will be a huge challenge, but it's definitely not impossible.

People who are impatient will also have a hard time with intermittent fasting because of what their expectations of the world happen to be. Impatient people expect the world to go fast, for things to be where they expect it *when* they expect it, and for progress to be made when they're ready for it to be made. In essence, impatient people are the opposite of productive intermittent fasters, for people skilled and practiced with IF know that patience is the ultimate virtue. It takes two weeks only to get fully past just the *detoxification* period for intermittent fasting, so clearly, impatient people will need those urges recalibrated before they're ready to handle the personal practice of consistency and waiting that gives life to the IF technique (and lifestyle).

Moody individuals will likely only see their emotional situations worsened by intermittent fasting, but these types of people often don't choose to fast intermittently because they want to fix their mood disorders. Instead, these people choose IF to lose weight, gain energy, fight aging, heal themselves or otherwise, and the emotional side-effects are just that. I recommend these individuals look at the bigger picture of intermittent fasting. This eating pattern and lifestyle change can make great waves in one's life that cause him or her to feel increasingly moody or troubled. By having increased awareness of the bigger picture, moody people might be able to hold off on transitioning to IF until they're healed enough to handle all the switch has to offer.

People who are excessively reserved or conservative in personality may find that intermittent fasting doesn't work for them because they struggle through the detox period and can't get any farther. It is true that the first two weeks of intermittent fasting – the detox period – are intense, both physically and emotionally. Sometimes, people break down into tears or have emotional explosions otherwise during this detoxification time, and overly reserved or conservative individuals will likely *not* appreciate being exposed to moments like this, much less that potential within their selves. If these types of people can learn to laugh at themselves and ride emotional waves more calmly, they'll have as much to gain from IF as any of the best of us.

Finally, when considering young people under the age of 18, we get back into physical traits and conditions a bit more than character traits, but it's undeniable that someone's youth makes it very difficult for intermittent fasting to work in his or her favor. No offense, but you're immature, and your body is even more immature, so you need all the available nutrients around you to help you grow properly. Limiting nutritional intake in any way (whether it's the *what* you eat or *when* it happens) will not be good for you until you're at least 18 and living your best life in that strong, fully-actualized, adult body.

Chapter 5: Different Methods of Intermittent Fasting

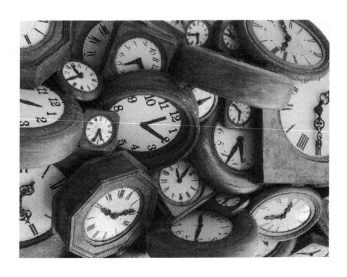

While there are many methods for intermittent fasting, only a handful of them works well specifically for women, and others work well for women in special cases. Overall, the goal is to learn about each method, its strengths, and its weaknesses, and then to choose which is right for you, given the current stage of your life and what struggles you face at the moment.

This chapter is dedicated to helping you through this complicated choosing process. In the following pages, ten methods for intermittent fasting will be discussed and compared according to their divergent results, difficulties, goals, and findings. Furthermore, their differences in complications and physical conditions will be analyzed for a true comparison to be achieved.

By the end of this chapter, you should feel almost overwhelmed with information about the different intermittent fasting styles, but you should also have a sense of being deeply grounded, for you will have a much better understanding of which method is right for you, or at least which method you'd like to start out trying! By the time you're done with the final page of this section, you should be empowered and ready to begin your own IF adventure.

Crescendo Method

The crescendo method of intermittent fasting is the one voted most productive for female-bodied practitioners. This method is well-known for its gentle approach to fasting, its caution, and awareness of hormonal balance, its ability to help you lose weight, and its gradual introduction (which works especially well for women with inconsistent work or life schedules).

Through the crescendo method, the individual will fast 12 to 16 hours at a time for two or three days a week that is not consecutive days. For instance, she might fast Sunday, normally eat Monday and Tuesday, fast Wednesday, normally eat Thursday, fast Friday, eat normally on Saturday, and repeat the pattern the next Sunday. During fast days, light cardio exercises or yoga can be practiced, but no intense workouts are allowed, due to the long hours involved in the fast. As needed, drink lots of water (with salt added if/when you get dizzy!) and coffee if you desire any energy boosts.

After two successful weeks of this pattern of fasting, additional days can be added, or the timing can be tweaked based on what's working and what isn't. This method amps up the power after the initial detoxification period, based on the abilities and reach of the individual. It builds in effect, but the impact remains the same such as increased health and decreased weight while respecting hormones and the potential for hefty mood swings.

Lean-Gains Method (14:10)

The lean-gains method has several different incarnations on the web, but its fame comes from the fact that it helps shed fat while building it into muscle almost immediately. Through the lean-gains method, you'll find yourself able to shift all that fat to be muscle through a rigorous practice of fasting, eating right, and exercising.

Through this method, you fast anywhere from 14 to 16 hours and then spend the remaining 10 or 8 hours each day engaged in eating and exercise. This method, as opposed to the crescendo, features daily fasting and eating, rather than alternated days of eating versus not. Therefore, you don't have to be quite so cautious about extending the physical effort to exercise on the days you are fasting because those days when you're fasting are literally every day!

For the lean-gains method, start fasting only 14 hours and work it up to 16 if you feel comfortable with it, but never forget to drink enough water and be careful about expending too much energy on exercise! Remember that you want to *grow* in health and potential through intermittent fasting. You'll certainly not want to lose any of that growth by forcing the process along.

16:8 Method

The 16:8 method of intermittent fasting is increasingly popular with practitioners of IF because it's often voted as the easiest one to enact. For women especially, this method is the logical extension of the lean-gains method, except it places less focus on intense physical exercise that would accompany the fasting.

With the 16:8 method of IF, you'll fast for 16 hours and then use the remaining 8-hour window to eat. Most people skip breakfast immediately upon waking and use their sleeping time to get that initial 16 hours of fasting together. Others will stop eating earlier in the night and then breakfast with their morning meal. Regardless, all the meals of the day will take place in the 8-hour eating window, which means you can probably fit three smaller meals into that time, but it can also mean that two meals might work better some days.

Overall, the 16:8 method is a great one to start with, especially if you sleep ten or more hours each night. If you're not sure which method to start with, try this one and then build up from it! Some people go from 16:8 to 20:4 while others use it as a diving board into alternate-day fasting. Try whatever works for you, but whatever you do, try!

20:4 Method

Stepping things up a notch from the 14:10 and 16:8 methods, the 20:4 method is a tough one to master, for it is rather unforgiving. People talk about this method of intermittent fasting as intense and highly restrictive, but they also say that the effects of living this method are almost unparalleled with all other tactics.

For the 20:4 method, you'll fast for 20 hours each day and squeeze all your meals, all your eating, and all your snacking into 4 hours. People who attempt 20:4 normally have two smaller meals or just one large meal and a few snacks during their 4-hour window to eat, and it really is up to the individual which four hours of the day they devote to eating.

The trick for this method is to make sure you're not over-eating or bingeing during those 4-hour windows to eat. It is all-too-easy to get hungry during the 20-hour fast and have that feeling then propel you into intense and unrealistic hunger or meal sizes after the fast period is over. Be careful if you try this method. If you're new to intermittent fasting, work your way up to this one gradually, and if you're working your way up already, only make the shift to 20:4 when you know you're ready. It would surely disappoint if all your progress with intermittent fasting got hijacked by one poorly thought-out goal with 20:4 method.

12:12 Method

As another of the easier methods of intermittent fasting, 12:12 method is well-suited to beginning practitioners. Many people actually live out 12:12 method without any forethought simply because of their sleeping and eating schedule but turning 12:12 into a conscious practice can have just as many positive effects on your life as the more drastic 20:4 method claims.

For this method, in particular, you fast for 12 hours and then enter a 12-hour eating window. It's not difficult whatsoever to get three small meals and several snacks, or two big meals and a snack into your day with this method. With 12:12, the standard meal timing works just fine. For instance, many of us already stop eating at 8 or 9 o'clock at night and then wait until 8 or 9 o'clock the next morning for breakfast. With this 12-hour gap between meals, these people are unintentionally already professionals at 12:12 method.

Ultimately, this method is a great one to start from, for a lot of variation can be built into this scheduling when you're ready to make things more interesting. Easily and without much effort, 12:12 can become 14:10 or even 16:8, and in seemingly no time, you can find yourself trying alternate-day or crescendo methods, too. Start with what's normal for you, and this method might be exactly that!

5:2 Method

When it comes to the intermittent fasting methods that have several hours each day set aside to fast and the lingering hours set aside to eat, something gets lost in translation. Some people come to intermittent fasting with aims at big lifestyle changes, or with hopes of experiencing whole new timing and relationships to food. In that case, these individuals might prefer 5:2 method.

Like the crescendo method, 5:2 goes back to several days "on" and several days a week "off" when it comes to fasting. In specific, this method of IF (being more extreme than any others we've looked at so far) involves a severe restriction of caloric intake for two days a week and regular feeding the remaining five days. On the two restricted-intake days, the practitioner is only allowed 500 calories per day to maintain and actualize the goals of the fast.

If you're having trouble making 5:2 method work, try a different style of intermittent fasting altogether. It could be that this strange on-and-off method doesn't suit your lifestyle, and there are clearly enough other options that there's bound to be *something* that works just right for *you*.

Eat-Stop-Eat (24 Hour) Method

This method of fasting is incredibly similar to the crescendo method. The only discernable difference is that there's no anticipation of increasing (of "crescendo-ing") into a more intense fasting pattern with time. For the eat-stop-eat method, you decide which days you want to take off from eating, and then you run with it until you've lost that weight and then you keep running with the lifestyle for good because you won't be able to imagine life without it.

The eat-stop-eat method involves one to two days a week being 100% oriented towards fasting, with the other five to six days concerning "business as normal." The one or two days spent fasting are then full 24-hour days spent without eating anything at all. During these days, of course, water and coffee are still fine to drink (in fact, anything is still acceptable to drink during fasting periods as long as it's not too thick like a smoothie or protein shake), but no food items can be consumed whatsoever. Exercise is also frowned upon on those fasting days but see what your body can handle before you decide how that should all work out.

Some people might start thinking they're using the crescendo method but end up sticking with eat-stop-eat. The two are so similar. It's easy to see how this situation might occur. Furthermore, some others work *up* to the eat-stop-eat method from 14:10 or 16:8 methods. It could be that these individuals tried the daily fast window technique and wanted something more intense. Clearly, this method qualifies!

Alternate-Day Method

The alternate-day method is admittedly a little confusing, but the reason it could be so confusing could come, in part, from how much wiggle room it provides for the practitioner. This method is great for people who don't have a consistent schedule or any sense of one, and it is therefore incredibly forgiving for those who don't quite have everything together for themselves yet.

When it comes down to it, alternate-day intermittent fasting is really up to you. You should try to fast every other day, but it doesn't have to be that precise. Similarly with crescendo method, as long as you fast two to three days a week, with a break day or two in between each fasting day, you're set! Basically then, you'll want to eat normally for three or four days out of each week, and when you encounter a fasting day, you don't even need to completely fast! I told you this diet was forgiving! All you need to do on these days is restrict your caloric intake to 20-25% of your standard intake (~500 calories total, each day).

Alternate-day fasting is a solid place to start from, especially if you work a varying schedule or still have yet to get used to a consistent one. If you want to make things more intense from this starting point, the alternate-day method can easily become the eat-stop-eat method, the crescendo method, or the 5:2 method. Essentially, this method is a great place to begin.

The Warrior Method

The warrior method is incredibly similar to 20:4 method, but with one major philosophical difference, which makes this method all that much more interesting. The warrior method takes as its philosophical base the experience of the hunter/gatherer ancestors we evolved from. It's as if this method looks back at the origins of intermittent fasting and tries to make its example as historically accurate as possible.

In sum, warrior method involves fasting for 20 hours a day (although you can have one cup of raw, fresh fruit and vegetables dispersed throughout that 20 hours) and then eating one large meal during the 4-hour feeding window. Just like the warrior coming home from the hunt, the individual practicing warrior method will spend most of the day working (i.e. the fast lasts all day). Only to come home and focus on one large meal (i.e. the 4-hour eating window would always take place during the evening), from which the body can then extract all its necessary nutrients and proteins for energy, alertness, and fat burning.

Warrior method is the logical extension of 20:4 method when you want to take things up a notch of intensity (or of philosophical rigor). It can also be scaled back to 16:8 or 14:10 easily if you notice things just aren't working with this method for you. The biggest danger of warrior method is overeating during that one meal. To help protect against problematic overeating, make sure to have that one cup of fruit or veg as a snack throughout your 20-hour fast, and you can even try breaking up your big meal into smaller sections that are eaten across the 4-hour feeding window if things still aren't working out. If these adjustments don't curb the overeating, another method would definitely suit you better.

Spontaneous Skipping Method

As the purposefully least-organized method of the bunch, spontaneous skipping method leaves most of the definition and planning to the individual. There's no easy division of time between fasting and feeding. There's no delineating of how much time needs to be spent on what. In fact, there are no standards for this plan whatsoever. The individual determines all this planning for him or herself.

In this case, all you need to do is skip one or two meals each day. That's all you need to do. Skip breakfast and your second snack one day, skip lunch and dinner the next (in favor of a bedtime snack), and then skip breakfast again the day after. Skip meals based on what's convenient for you, too!

If you're someone who has trouble defining a daily schedule, if you're someone who balks at routine, or if you're someone who works increasingly varying shifts at work; this intermittent fasting method is probably perfect for you. Try this one out to start or try it after you've realized some of the more "structured" methods don't work, based on your lifestyle. Regardless of how you do it, just try it! Even if you're not fully working at intermittent fasting quite yet, dip your toes in the water! Skip a meal here and then, and I promise, your body will thank you for it.

Which Method Suits Which Woman & Which Lifestyle Best

While there are ten methods for intermittent fasting listed here, there are numerous others in existence, and the ultimate truth for which method works best for you comes from within you. *You* are the one who can tell if things are working out or need to be changed, but if you aren't sure, you should definitely be in touch with a personal or family doctor to be sure you're not unknowingly doing damage while you're trying to heal yourself and lose that pesky weight.

Amongst the tens of options for intermittent fasting methods, there are a few that are more geared towards supporting female anatomy, hormones, and health. The ones that fit this description are methods crescendo, eat-stop-eat, alternate-day, and 5:2. Ultimately, these four are better-suited for women's health, but when it comes down to which one suits *you* best, consider the following qualifications.

Consider your lifestyle. When you decide on which method of IF to use, think of when you normally wake up in the morning as well as how much sleep you normally get. Think of how often you work and what hours of the day they cover and don't forget to consider whether or not you can eat freely at work! That flexibility (or rigidity) will be pivotal in helping you decide whether you should do full days of fasting or have eating windows dispersed throughout every day. In fact, if you *can't* eat at work, you could plan to use that time as part of your daily fast hours! Furthermore, think of the times of day you normally get hungry and build your IF schedule around those needs! You don't have to be forced to suffer or starve whatsoever while working with intermittent fasting. Help your future self by using your strengths and pre-determined routines and applying them to your IF method and scheduling. You'll thank yourself later.

Consider your abilities and your body. How long can you really go without eating? Have you tried fasting of any kind before? Are you familiar with using any sort of dietary restriction to increase your health? Also, what's your current diet like? Are you already exposed to whole foods, packed with good nutrients, or are you eating a largely processed diet? All of these factors determine how your transition into the intermittent fast will look. For instance, if you're eating largely processed foods, you might be a little more irritable and stinky (literally!) when you proceed through the detoxification period. If you're already familiar with fasting, you might have a higher tolerance for hunger waves, so 5:2 might be better for you than 16:8. If you're unfamiliar with restricting your diet whatsoever, you might be better off starting with a loosely-defined plan such as spontaneous skipping method before trying a more rigorous and demanding style of intermittent fasting.

Consider your family and friends. When you decide which method to start with, you'll have to ponder how strong the influences of others around you happen to be. How independent are you, and how much do you feel you control your own life and make your own choices? Who do you normally hang out with and, more importantly, how often do your engagements involve food? How much influence does your family have over you, your health, and your weight? Are they healthful and like-minded, or do they stress you out to the point where you can't consider being healthy whatsoever in their presence? Think seriously about the people in your life and how they'll influence your fasting schedule. If you're concerned what others will think, choose a method where you can eat at more "normal" times and join them without standing out. If you're unperturbed by these considerations, go for whatever feels right otherwise!

From these three considerations, you should be able to discern which method or methods are safe, and from what places you can begin. As always, do your proper research, speak with your doctor, and trust yourself. If things aren't going well, you'll feel it, so never be afraid to tweak things if they're not working right. If you've chosen to work with intermittent fasting, it becomes your responsibility to take care of your body in relation to its changes after IF. If you're ready to fast, you better be ready and conscious enough to start healing. That way, your future is bright no matter what pitfalls might lead you astray along the way. That way, your health is in your own hands, and that's really what matters.

Chapter 6: How to Get Started

At this point, you likely know which intermittent fasting strategy you're going to employ or which ones you're going to try deciding between since there truly *are* so many options, so it's time to start thinking of how to put your plan into action. While intermittent fasting can seem, to some, much less daunting than an entire diet change, it is just as intense as becoming vegan from being a meat-eater for others. That being said, no matter which camp you fall into, you'll likely need a few pointers for the adjustment period.

The gist of this chapter is to give you the information you need to make the transition into your first (or next) intermittent fast as easy and painless as it can be. You'll be provided with tips to help establish a new routine as well as informational tidbits of what to expect, what to do and what not to do, what to look out for and, for worst-case scenario moments, when to quit.

Before the chapter is finished, you will also be guided through common mistakes in the transition to intermittent fast. The hope is that you'll then be able to avoid such instances in your own experience as you decide how and when to move forward with IF yourself. You'll also be exposed to ways to "protect" against potential hiccups in the plan. Simply put, the more forethought, the better; the more you're mentally and emotionally ready for, the more successful your adventure with intermittent fasting will be overall. Let's make our way into getting started!

Transitional Tips

When you're about to begin your process of intermittent fasting, you'll need to have a few tricks up your sleeve to make the transition as painless as possible, and that's what this section is all about. First of all, make sure you do have some sort of method planned. Pick that plan and stick with it, at least for the first week. Next, do any extra research you may need to do, considering your body type and any diseases or disorders that you may have. This extra bit of research may be game-changing for you, in terms of making sure your transition into IF has no disruptions or toxic effects for your body type. If it's necessary at this point, check with your doctor to ensure that you're on the right track and that the method you've chosen poses no harm to you.

Something else you can do before start IF, is to look at your diet ahead of time and adjust things to be a little easier. As I mentioned before, a diet composed of primarily processed foods may pose complications for the individual during the detoxification period. As you can, start to replace processed foods, with whole foods (fruits, vegetables, grains, nuts, seeds, etc.) that support your health and healing. Additionally, as you plan which method you'll undertake, you can go into more detail and make sure your feasting is packed with the right nutrients between fast periods. Calculate the calories you'll need for each fast, the macronutrients you'll need to refuel, and the training you anticipate you'll be able to handle. The more forethought, the better.

When it comes to that first day of getting started in the intermittent fast lifestyle, the following pieces of advice will help to make things flow with ease. First of all, on the evening before, don't eat a late dinner, and don't eat after dinner. Make sure to have lots of drinks on hand for the fasting process ahead. Healthy and IF-safe drinks are listed above in chapter 3 for your convenience. Imagine that night before that you're beginning your fast at sundown or after that early dinner. Then, when you go to sleep and wake up in the morning, you've already done almost 12 hours of fasting. At that point, delay your breakfast the next morning, and you can easily achieve 12 hours if not 14 of fasting right off the bat.

During this waiting period, have as many IF-safe drinks as needed, and then, when the eating window comes (if you choose a method that involves an eating window or at least if you try this day-1 transition guide), engage in eating, but don't snack too much. The following days, whether they involve eating windows or not, try to cut out snacks more often to help your body adjust. Other things you can do before and during your transition to IF include skipping breakfasts habitually or simply delaying them, having earlier dinners, or substituting snacks for smoothies.

Help for Routine-Setting

After the first few days, you may need a little help getting the routine affirmed and established, and the following pieces of advice are attuned to help with that exact problem. To assist in routine-setting, remember to keep things slow and simple, especially at the beginning of your process. Don't push yourself too hard and keep your expectations for the fast (and on yourself) realistic and grounded.

If things aren't working out, go back to your considerations from the method-selection section of chapter 5 and check that you've chosen a method that actually aligns with your strengths. It could be that you've tried to start with a method that's too disruptive of your standard routine. It's much more productive to transition into something that's a somewhat "logical" extension of your daily activities.

What to Expect

When you begin intermittent fasting, there are several things you should expect from your experience, regardless of whether they're helpful or not. The points below will walk you through those details to prepare you for what's to come.

First of all, mornings may be completely different for you. You will likely find that your mornings become filled with energy or completely lethargic, depending on whether you were a morning or night person beforehand. Furthermore, you may experience your worst hunger pangs during the morning time, but this element is also affected by whether you're a morning or night person. Finally, coffee will become your best friend, if it's not already. Mornings may be the most serious times of fasting for you, and even if they're not fasting periods, you're still going to need that infamous morning juice (coffee, or at least something caffeinated that similarly kick-starts metabolism) to get you through the day as it is now, with less food in it.

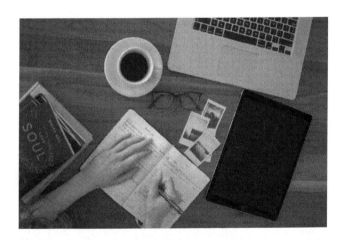

Certain things will increase. During your initial transition period into intermittent fasting, your abilities to plan and organize are liable to massively and noticeably increase. You might find that scheduling your fast into your week feels impossible before you begin, but after the first few days, it will become more second-nature to organize and think in this way. Additionally, you will almost certainly become more mindful of the world around you, of your internal feelings, and of how food truly affects you. As one final note, recall all the potential benefits of intermittent fasting. Go back to chapter 3 and explore the "pros" category of the chapter's first section. Remind yourself of what you're working to grow in yourself, and you're sure to be propelled through the hard times.

Other things will decrease. The most common goal of intermittent fasting is to lose weight (yay!), and that will almost assuredly happen for every IF practitioner. That weight is bound to decrease with the appropriate application of intermittent fasting and healthy diet, given your body type and physical needs. Furthermore, you may lose sleep, at least during the first two weeks' detoxification period, which is detailed more in the next paragraph. Although sleep may be difficult, it will settle back into a normal pattern, and if you always have troubles with sleep, you might even find that you have the easiest, most restful sleep of your life while you're intermittently fasting.

During a period of the first two or so weeks, you will definitely go through a detoxification period. You will get stinky, moody, cranky, and tired. You will feel weird bursts of energy and then nothing at all. If you're working out as you practice intermittent fasting, you might find that your workouts during the first two weeks are especially exhausting or unproductive. You might have an emotional moment or two, but after these first two weeks, those powerful side-effects should go away, for they're all a part of the detox associated with the transition. You have to get through the rough patch to reap the rewards, however, so stick with the process and fight through those crunchy, harsh times. You'll be thankful you pushed through, no matter how smelly you may get.

You may also experience somewhat negative side-effects, which will be detailed further in the section titled "What to Lookout For," which appears later in this chapter.

Finally, your relationship with food will become entirely different. It may take a couple of days — it may even take the entire detox period to get it right to settle into eating the *right amount* during your eating windows. At first, you might have trouble with either eating too much or not enough when it's time to eat, but you will be urged to work through any food dependency issues by this process regardless of how often and how much you eat. During times of fast, one can't help but consider with new eyes how food, hunger, and hangry feelings affect one's relationship with others and the world.

What to Do/What Not to Do

When it comes down to it, knowing concisely what to do and what not to do will be the informational backbone to your success with intermittent fasting.

What to do includes:

- Start slow

- Track your progress

- Live normally, otherwise
    - Especially in times of fast, work and play are especially distracting when you're hungry!

- Help to suppress hunger with drinks like mineral water and with gum

- Keep tabs on your hormonal health
    - As a woman, it is especially important that you perform this work to troubleshoot IF in your life.

- Focus on fats when you eat (*without* making fat consumption your main goal)

On the other hand, **what not to do** includes:

- Don't start too hard and fast
    - Ease into it!

- Don't give up after just a week

- o This is a big no-no unless you display warning signs and worst-case-scenario markers.

- Don't diet too fiercely

- Don't work out too much

- Don't continue to intermittently fast even after you display warning signs

- Don't constantly eat during the eating windows
  - o Don't forget that your body still needs breaks in eating to digest!

What to Lookout For

As you engage with intermittent fasting, there may be warning signs that your body is not benefitting from the process at hand. You'll have to be very keen and conscious of these warning signs, for if they appear, alterations will need to be made if your success and health are the goals (as they should be!). Overall, look out for warning signs like constant headaches, tiredness without the ability to sleep, dizziness, lightheadedness, or constant sleeping. While some of these elements can be signals that adjustments in the process are all that's needed, if you had any of these problems before trying IF and they've gotten *worse* as you continued with IF, you may have reached a quitting point. Talk to your doctor if you come up against any of these warning signs, or you can even go back to section 1 of chapter 3 in this eBook to help troubleshoot these "cons" of the experience.

Something else to look out for includes those general hunger pangs, but as we've discussed before, just make sure to ride those urges out like waves, for they surely will pass. Check in with yourself mentally and emotionally as you proceed with intermittent fasting, too, for your knowledge of yourself will be the most helpful aspect of making sure that your process is healthy for you. If you notice that your personality starts to align with those problematic traits from chapter 4, try scaling down the intensity of your fast, or you could also try processing those personality traits and rescaling them to be appropriate and more health-oriented. The process of intermittent fasting is one that can be easily abused and twisted into something that's unhealthy, but the better you know yourself, and the more you seek growth in this effort, the better off you'll be when it comes to IF.

When to Quit

Since you're female, you are a bit more likely to experience worst-case-scenario intermittent fasting moments than a male would be, but when you do come up against these scenarios, do not doubt that it is truly time for you to stop. Pushing beyond this point means your life stands at risk, and no fitness regime is worth that price. Do not take these worst-case-scenario warnings lightly.

Worst-case-scenario warnings include:

- Burning in the pit of your stomach
  - This sensation is a likely sign of gastritis or something even worse.

- Vomiting even when you've hardly eaten
  - You could have gastric irritation, an imbalance of electrolytes, or something more dangerous.

- Fainting

- o This issue is especially worrisome if it becomes habitual.

- Feeling a pain in your stomach or chest

- Experiencing diarrhea
  - o Diarrhea is troubling because can contribute to dehydration and imbalance of electrolytes if not noticed and fixed in time.

- Worrying period symptoms
  - o such as: complete loss of period, excessive bleeding, or spotting when you're not supposed to be

Most Common Mistakes & How to Avoid Them

In order to avoid these warning signs and to be able to continue without having to quit or recalibrate too intensely, glance over the following section of common mistakes. With the information at your fingertips, you should be able to avoid these pitfalls expertly and therefore succeed in your IF ventures. Whoever said it hurt to learn from others' mistakes? That's right, no one. Generally, the most common mistakes with intermittent fasting are as follows: eating incorrectly, stopping too eagerly, spending fast time incorrectly, or forcing things to happen.

When it comes to eating incorrectly, there are a few subpoints to note. Sometimes, people overeat when they breakfast or breakfast too harshly, while others don't eat enough. Some others still simply eat the wrong foods and put their bodies at a detriment. Others on top of that forget the importance (and necessity) of drinking enough liquids, even during fast times.

These common mistakes are easily avoided, however. To combat the mistakes of this nature, plan out your meals better! Think of portion size, calories, and macronutrients in the foods you're about to eat, and arrange your meals to support health. Furthermore, you can eat slower if you find yourself eating too much, or at least make sure you have time to eat enough if you haven't been. Reconsider your weekly menus, make sure you're drinking liquids, and pace yourself! Even though it can *feel like* you're starving, you're just fine, and the food is there for you when it's time to eat. You'll get the hang of it in time.

The mistake of stopping too eagerly can be avoided by simply being as patient as possible with the process. Take it one week at a time, but always have your eye on the horizon where intermittent fasting is accepted into your life as a healthy and productive lifestyle arrangement. If you mess up, that's okay! Don't give up entirely; just push through the moment and keep the energy going. If you slip up, you don't have to stop. If the method isn't working, you don't have to stop either. Troubleshoot and keep going. Be patient and see what IF can do for your life.

The mistake of spending fast time incorrectly can put you in situations where you're accidentally hanging out around food during the fasting window. You could end up fasting when you're at work when your place of work involves food. You could spend it thinking about food rather than doing the things that are necessary for your health. Try to think in advance with intermittent fasting. Plan your days to be busy during the fast time. Think of where you'll be and who you'll be with. Protect yourself against pressuring food situations too. This mistake is easily avoided with proper forethought.

The mistake of forcing things to happen can involve imposing your timing to be perfect, making yourself stop trying with a simple slip-up, setting unrealistic training and exercise goals, or otherwise. Rather than put yourself in situations that feel forced or experiences that need to be "corrected" with force, make sure to take things slowly but much more importantly, allow your first week of intermittent fasting to be as low-expectation as possible. Try not to have any workout goals. Try not to have any weight loss goals. Just try to focus on the food and the waiting; when to eat, when to fast, what you feel during each period, and what your body feels capable of doing around this patient work. By attuning more to your body and its actual abilities, you're much less likely to have to force anything in the future, for your decisions and schedule will have been designed with those base and realistic capabilities in mind.

Protecting Against Potential Roadblocks & Hiccups

While you proceed with your first (or next) attempts at intermittent fasting, there are a few things you can keep in mind to ensure you don't get snagged up on potential roadblocks and hiccups, of which there are several. Those common mistakes and warning signs certainly count as "roadblocks and hiccups," too, so by learning and internalizing the information provided in this chapter, you're already one step ahead of the game in that you're already armed with the knowledge necessary to keep yourself protected.

Overall, there are two big things you can do to protect yourself:

(1) Remember your purpose with intermittent fasting whether it's:

- weight loss and maintenance,
- the goal of avoiding medication with a disease you currently suffer,
- the prevention of future disease,
- general longevity in this life,
- or something else entirely.

(2) Think *past and through* what makes you nervous. For example,

- try not to be overly hopeful and excited with the possibilities IF provides,
- don't let yourself get hung up on worries about your metabolism,
- try not to get distracted about concerns about whether skipping snacking and breakfast is OK,
- don't let yourself get caught up over a few stubborn pounds,
- and overall – basically, don't sweat the small stuff.

Do the research, feel hopeful, and remember your goals. As long as you keep these points in mind, even if you do meet a roadblock, it won't be the *end* of the road, for you'll be much more eager and willing to disassemble the roadblock so you can move forward freely.

Chapter 7: Intermittent Fasting for the Overworked & Stressed-Out Woman

At this point, you surely have a solid foundation of knowledge about intermittent fasting under your belt, and you likely have decided on whether or not you'll attempt IF yourself. If you decided that IF *is* right for you, the method that's best for you has probably been settled upon at this juncture. Now comes the serious part.

There are times in a woman's life when intermittent fasting creates certain issues that need to be addressed with alterations to the fast, its length, or its strictness. For women who lead very stressed-out or overworked lives, intermittent fasting can be both helpful and hurtful but only if not practiced in the correct, most health-oriented ways. This chapter is dedicated to hashing out intermittent fasting's effects on everyday and long-term stress. It will explore how you can add IF to your life alongside daily stress without making things worse, and it will provide details on what foods and IF methods are best-suited for healing in your case.

By the end of this chapter, you should be confident that you can move forward with intermittent fasting despite stresses in your life. If you have anxiety, if you have a demanding work life, if you are often stressed-out, intermittent fasting can still be right for you! In fact, IF can even help people who lead high-stress lifestyles. It all depends on the approach.

IF & Its Effects on Stress

It is true that intermittent fasting poses a certain "stress" to the individual's system, but it does so in the same way that exercise works on the body. The trick for both is appropriate and health application and dosage. The next section will provide information on what application and dosages are appropriate for women, depending on how much stress they experience, but this section concerns the science of how intermittent fasting decreases stress to each practitioner on the cellular level.

Bodily "stress" as we feel it, regarding anxiety and frustrations, is triggered by the hormone cortisol, and intermittent fasting itself does *not* decrease that stress response in the body. What it *does* do is decrease the stress our *cells* experience as they age and deal with chronic disease. This type of stress is called oxidative stress, and it occurs when free radical molecules, which are unstable and problematic, interact with and do damage to the body's more important molecules, such as proteins and DNA.

A study conducted in 2005 on rodents and monkeys, and then another conducted in 2007 on human asthma patients, revealed that intermittent fasting might help make our cells more resistant to oxidative stress as well as inflammations within the body. Scientifically, these are the same effects as we discussed in chapter 3 with the "pros" of intermittent fasting. The 2005 study additionally reveals how intermittent fasting even acts on the brain in ways that could decrease depression on the long-term for practitioners!

Essentially, these studies reveal how intermittent fasting makes the body oriented to work against aging and disease, to jolt itself back to life, and to remember how to heal itself. Given this effect *in* the body, it may be true that intermittent fasting doesn't help with overall stress, but it does work to heal things internally in a way that eases overall stress over time, depending on your situation, your personality, and how often you choose to fast.

How to Start Without Adding More Stress

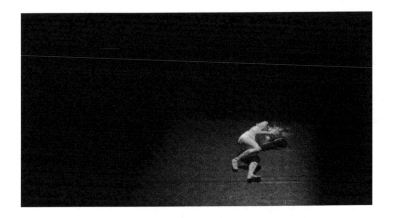

If you experience intense stress periodically, daily, or chronically, you will have a unique relationship with intermittent fasting. I cannot lie, this practice of patterned timing with eating *will* add a degree of stress to your day. Following an extra routine, being sure to get the right calories, eating at the right times, etc., all these details will add to your tensions, but at the same time, the right application of the practice can be calming and affirming as you move forward. It can even be healing, as we learned with the 2005 rodent and monkey study.

The key is to remember that fasting is not the end-all, be-all answer to heal your stress. When applied to your life one or two weeks a month, IF can provide a healthy *jolt* to your cells and system overall. However, if you are a chronically stressed individual, when you start keep your demands on yourself with IF low (if you even choose to attempt it). If you do though, the final section of this chapter can guide you in which method works best for your experience.

For others who are not chronically stressed but perhaps daily or periodically, you may not have as hard a time with intermittent fasting, and it will certainly work to heal your cells bit by bit if you practice the right method for your situation (again, see the final section for your answers). To incorporate IF into your routine without adding more stress, start by using day-by-day fasting methods instead of eating-window, daily methods. Once you settle into a day-by-day method that feels right, you can see what 16:8 or 14:10 feels like as long as your body approves.

Finally, for those who experience no restriction due to a relative lack of stress in their lives, you won't really have to worry about using a specific method to avoid excess stress. For you, just go back to those basic considerations from the end of chapter 5 to choose the method that feels least stressful for you. If you're looking for a high-energy routine that *does* stress you out, so to speak, then go ahead and choose in that respect. The final section of this chapter will provide answers for you, too.

Best Foods & Drinks to Incorporate

For people who experience a lot of stress whether periodically, daily, or chronically, it may be the case that now isn't the right time for you to try intermittent fasting. On the other hand, you might want to try it just a day or two a week and learn more about nutrition in the meantime. This section will be of great help to people in your situation, for it will provide some quick and easy facts about the foods and drinks you can incorporate to de-stress and emotionally or mentally de-clutter your life.

Asparagus is naturally high in folate, which helps one stay calm amongst stressors.

Avocado is high in glutathione, vitamins E & B, folate, beta-carotene, and lutein, all of which help you stay immune to stress.

Beans are a great source of magnesium, which helps with any body aches associated with working out or fasting as well as reverse the effects of stress by regulating blood pressure and cortisol, and they're also relatively high in tryptophan, which increases serotonin in the brain and enhances mood.

Berries are incredibly high in antioxidants as well as vitamin C, which lowers blood pressure and levels of cortisol, the body's stress hormone.

Brown Rice is a great source of magnesium, which helps with any body aches associated with working out or fasting as well as reverse the effects of stress by regulating blood pressure and cortisol.

Carrots are high in beta-carotene but crunching away at a raw carrot can also be relaxing, just like chewing on ice – only healthier and much better for your teeth.

Chocolate, dark chocolate, in particular, increases serotonin (which makes for better moods) and decreases cortisol (that pesky stress hormone); it can also help lower blood pressure due to the powerful antioxidants present in this tasty treat.

Fatty Fish like salmon is great for helping with stress because it's high in omega-3s, and it's also relatively high in tryptophan, which increases serotonin in the brain and enhances mood.

Garlic is high in antioxidants and helps to neutralize those free radicals that cause oxidative stress on our cells. Garlic heals both types of "stress"!

Grass-Fed Beef is a great source of vitamins C, B, E, and beta-carotene, and it's also packed with omega-3s while being relatively low in fat.

Leafy Greens are high in magnesium, which helps with any body aches associated with working out or fasting as well as reverse the effects of stress by regulating blood pressure and cortisol, and they're also filled with healthy fiber!

Milk (*not as a drink during fast but with meals*) is high in vitamins D & B and is a great source of protein to combat stress' effects in the body.

Nuts are high in omega-3s as well as potassium and zinc, which makes them a great immunity booster against stresses of all kinds. They are also relatively high in tryptophan, which increases serotonin in the brain and enhances mood.

Oatmeal is a great source of fiber and helps to boost energy through its grainy potential, and oats are also relatively high in tryptophan, which increases serotonin in the brain and enhances mood.

Oranges are high in vitamin C, which helps strengthen one's stress response.

Oysters are an incredible source of zinc, which boosts one's immunity, protecting against all sorts of future stress.

Probiotics (*drink during fast & with meals; eat with meals too*) are unparalleled in their abilities to mitigate anxiety and alleviate stress levels. They can even enhance one's mood.

Red Peppers are high in vitamin C, which helps strengthen one's stress response.

Seeds are a great source of in magnesium, which helps with any body aches associated with working out or fasting as well as reverse the effects of stress by regulating blood pressure and cortisol, and they're also relatively high in tryptophan, which increases serotonin in the brain and enhances mood.

Soy Beans, whether eaten as edamame, tofu, or miso, are relatively high in tryptophan, which increases serotonin in the brain and enhances mood. When fermented in miso, soybeans become probiotic, which makes them work to block stress all the better!

Teas (*drink during fast & with meals) of all kinds help the drinker de-stress through lowered cortisol in the body. Even caffeinated teas, such as black tea, were able to decrease the stress response for many drinkers. More commonly, however, decaf teas do the trick faster with less potential to fail. Try chamomile, green, peppermint, or ginger teas to soothe and heal from within against more than just stress.

Turkey is packed with tryptophan, which increases serotonin in the brain and enhances mood as well as makes you feel sleepy after eating so much of it on Thanksgiving or Christmas day.

<u>Whole Wheat</u> provides a great energy boost as well as demonstrates a perfect source of fiber to keep the body running in tip-top shape.

<u>Yogurt</u>, like milk, is high in vitamins B & D as well as protein to help combat the effects of stress on one's body. Most yogurts are also probiotic!

Best Fasting Method for You

For the generally unstressed woman, the crescendo method is a great place to start, but really, any method can work well for you to help decrease stress and increase overall healing. If you want an extra challenge, try 20:4. This method will certainly give you something to work for!

For the periodically stressed-out woman, try starting with the crescendo method, but if you like, you can alter your plans and try methods 5:2, alternate-day, or eat-stop-eat. These methods seem to have more balance between structure and flexibility, while crescendo requires a little more vigor than this individuals' other approved methods will.

For the daily stressed-out woman, the ideal method for intermittent fasting will be something that's fairly low-maintenance and low-stress to begin with. Through alternate-day, 5:2, and eat-stop-eat, these individuals should be able to use meal skipping to ease into day-by-day fasting (rather than eating-window, which can be more anxiety-inducing for these types of people).

Finally, for the chronically stressed-out woman, the ideal method, if you should choose to pursue intermittent fasting at all, will be one that hardly demands forethought. Spontaneous skip method is absolutely best-suited for this type of individual, but if that style of intermittent fasting seems to work well and the individual wants more of a challenge, he or she can easily switch to 5:2 method and practice it only one or two weeks a month to start.

Chapter 8: Intermittent Fasting for the Breastfeeding Woman

One of the most heated debates in the field of intermittent fasting for women is whether or not it's productive for breastfeeding mothers to engage in intermittent fasting after their babies are born. People tend to feel strongly about their opinions in this debate, but it still comes down to what feels right for you.

If you're skimming through this section as someone who will have babies in the future, just let the ideas settle in and simmer. If you're reading through this book as a pregnant woman, read through these ideas but be sure to ask your doctor before you fully settle either way and make sure to do your rounds of research based on your body type and needs.

This chapter will be dedicated to hashing out the arguments in the field, and it will settle in a neutral stance that both reveals the dangers and the methods that have worked for breastfeeding IF mothers. Ultimately, the chapter will culminate on two sections about diet, the first informing about the standards for eating right while breastfeeding and the second providing five recipes to use in your personal life for health while breastfeeding.

By the end of this section, you should still be a little curious. You might have settled on whether or not you think breastfeeding while intermittent fasting is healthy, but you are likely still questioning. That's great, if so! Take those questions to the internet, to encyclopedias, or your to doctor and do the hard work to find out what's right for you. Your body and your baby will be forever thankful you did.

The Arguments in the Field: A Good Idea or Not?

When it comes down to the arguments in the field, there are two main camps. Some people think it's fine for mothers to intermittently fast while they're breastfeeding as long as they're following the right guidelines. Other people think it would be abhorrent for a mother even to consider intermittent fasting while she's breastfeeding. Of course, with there being two camps, these ideas demonstrate extremes along a binary, and the best method with extremes of this nature is finding their balance. Therefore, let your balance be established within this ongoing debate, and use the information provided to make the best decision for yourself, your body, and your baby.

In the "Yes" camp of individuals who think you can balance breastfeeding and intermittent fasting, the main argument is that it's only an *intermittent* fast! This group of individuals tends to think that of course, a woman can balance breastfeeding and intermittent fasting mostly because every woman, every pregnancy, and every case is different, so of course, every woman would consult her doctor to check and make sure things were okay before actually moving forward with the decision. These people also consider that you should compare your pregnancy goals to your personal goals, and if you'd rather focus on the latter, you maybe needn't breastfeed whatsoever! The arguments then fragment out from this group's main ideas into themes such as "Yes, IF and breastfeeding can be balanced *if* it's a short fast," "...*if* it's a less intense fast," or "...*if* it's a different diet to compensate." Regardless, the point is the same; you *absolutely can* plan an intermittent fast that doesn't interfere too much with your breastfeeding or your baby's health.

In the "No" camp of individuals who think you should never try to balance breastfeeding and intermittent fasting, the main argument is that you're removing your abilities to produce milk, which are so essential for the child and its growth overall. These people see that fewer nutrients will be contained in the milk when the mother consumes fewer nutrients, and they know that milk production itself can decrease when mothers restrict caloric intake. Furthermore, these individuals think that you shouldn't force things (by intermittent fasting) and that you should just ride with nature's punches until breastfeeding is over. It's just six months of waiting, after all, they say. These individuals would ask the breastfeeding mother to consider her intentions when she chooses to restrict food intake during this time. If her goals are motivated by others' opinions, whether of beauty, of what's "natural," or of timing, she is encouraged to question what *she* actually wants *for herself* and the baby, what's actually healthy, and what she's doing rushing things in the first place.

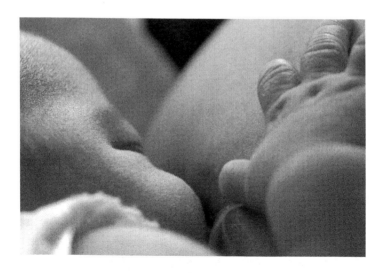

Possible Dangers

The possible dangers of combining intermittent fasting with breastfeeding are as follows:

- ## Less Milk! No Milk!

Yes, the breastfeeding mother will produce less milk when she restricts her caloric intake. This issue can be helped by fasting incredibly rarely and with lowered fast hours, less exercise, and less intensity of food restriction during eating periods. This danger is only legitimate for the mother who truly wants to *breast*feed her child consistently as the child's only source of food.

- ## No Energy!

Yes, the breastfeeding mother will have less energy for herself and to pay close attention to her baby if she's restricting caloric intake through intermittent fasting and still able to breastfeed her child for every meal. As long as the mother has a capable and non-disabled partner willing to pick up the slack and pay close attention to everything else, this might still be okay. Frequent check-ups to the doctor will ensure that this low energy level isn't detrimental to mama and baby's health.

- ## If you're sick, it will only make things worse!

Yes, it is true that if the breastfeeding mother is sick on top of everything else, intermittent fasting will exacerbate the problem to a dangerous degree for both mama and baby. In these cases, the mother should completely cease intermittent fasting until the sickness is gone. If she continues, her health and her baby's life are at risk.

- Other concerns: Anemia, Low Blood Pressure or Sugar, etc.

Sometimes, the pregnant mother might have health problems that are made worse through pregnancy and strained even further through the process of intermittent fasting. This reality is the primary reason why you should always check with your doctor before you choose to breastfeed and intermittently fast at the same time. Only your doctor knows all your tics and diseases, so only she will be able to make sure you're making the best choice for yourself and your family.

What Methods Have Worked

The methods that have worked to combine and balance intermittent fasting with breastfeeding are as follows:

- Low-Intensity Crescendo Method

Because crescendo method begins with just a few days a week, and those days aren't even full fast days, breastfeeding mothers might be able to work from this starting place to see if things are going to work out with IF at this time or not. If three days a week of basically 16:8 method, then go down to two days. If two days are still too much, go down to one day. If one day then feels good, stay there. If you feel like you can do more, try upping the ante to two days or going back to three days at 14:10 or 12:12 instead. There are ways to make this work!

- Flexible, Spontaneous Meal Skipping

The breastfeeding mother can work with intermittent fasting as long as the plan isn't too structured and restrictive. The most productive method for the woman in this position will be a very flexible spontaneous skip method. Whenever the mother has fully fed her child and feels lingering energy, she might try skipping her next meal. She might try skipping breakfast daily or cutting out a snack or two. Non-severe restrictions of this nature can be beneficial to both mama and baby, but they do have to be entirely *non-severe.*

- One Week out of the Month

One other method mama can try, is to "fast" only one week each month. Maybe she can try going throughout the month as it begins and waits until the last week of the month to see if she feels well and strong enough to produce milk and maintain an intermittent fast. In these cases, the best fasting strategy for that one week might be alternate-day or 5:2. However, 14:10 or 12:12 in that week might work just as well if not better for a breastfeeding mom. As always, see what works best for you with slow and flexible experimentation to start.

- Eventually...

Another method that can work is, with lack of a better name idea, the "Eventually..." method, whereby the breastfeeding mother realizes that she *can* intermittently fast once the child is six months old. Some scholars really think that the baby should have mother's milk for the first six months, but that afterward, it doesn't matter so much. Moms can easily piggyback on this logic by riding out the first six months with the baby and *then* switching to start balancing intermittent fasting with breastfeeding when that time is up, and the need to have breastmilk is lessened for the newborn.

- Overall Tips

Overall, if you do decide to intermittently fast while breastfeeding, keep these five tips in mind. First, hydrate! Hydrate to an excessive degree almost, but make sure you're getting a good mix of water, electrolytes, teas, and more. Just water all the time will make you feel faint, dizzy, or lightheaded, none of which are productive whatsoever.

Second, take supplements! Breastfeeding mothers should be getting a variety of nutrients through several sources. If you're intermittent fasting while breastfeeding, one thing you can do to troubleshoot is to take supplements to replace what's being missed or overlooked. Supplements of great necessity are vitamins B1, B2, B6, and B12, choline, vitamins A & D, selenium, iodine, folate, calcium, iron, copper, and zinc.

Third, you don't *have* to lose that baby weight intermittently fast! Try exercising consistently instead. Try dieting instead. You don't have to stop eating or engage in a pattern like that to lose weight. There are several other things and practices to try to shed post-partum weight. Don't think that IF is the only option and remember, you can always come back to IF in six months when the baby is older.

Fourth, you can try out intermittent fasting and breastfeeding and use your baby's diaper evidence to see if it's healthy for the child or not. Is the baby's stool runny? It should be! If it becomes solid, you're not getting enough liquids through your body. If it's an abnormal color, something might be up. Check with your doctor if your child's waste looks anything other than normal, for it might be a clue that your intermittent fasting isn't helping at all but rather hurting.

Fifth, no matter what you've decided for your intermittent fast at this time, if you feel or notice any of those warning signs or worst-case-scenario markers, *eat something.* Your goals to fast are not more important than your baby's and your health. Remember that you're a mother as well as an individual; now more than ever, it's important not to push yourself past the breaking point.

Eating Right While Breastfeeding

Making sure you get the right nutrients for your baby while you're breastfeeding, especially IF breastfeeding, is essential! This section will go through facts about different foods and drinks that will be beneficial to your health and the baby's as you attempt breastfeeding, with or without the addition of intermittent fasting. You will learn how to eat smart to help with postpartum weight loss, how to behave in ways that help you lose weight, how to eat without affecting your milk supply, and more.

Avocados are high in healthy fats as well as vitamins B, K, C, & E. Furthermore, avocados are high in potassium and folates that help the breastfeeding mother produce more milk while keeping her body and heart healthy.

Beans & Legumes provide vitamins, minerals, phytoestrogens, and protein! They're great for breastfeeding mothers, especially when a variety of beans and legumes are eaten, for they enable the mother to produce a constantly healthy milk supply.

Blueberries have lots of vitamins and minerals that keep your energy level high through their complex carbohydrates. They're also high in antioxidants to keep you healthy and glowing for baby!

Brown Rice is a great addition to your diet while breastfeeding, for it grants the calories needed and it's known to make good-quality milk for babies. These healthy carbs are just what you need.

Eggs, being high in protein, provide fatty acids for your milk and energy for your*self*.

Fish like salmon is high in a healthy fat called DHA as well as being low in mercury. If you're looking for protein, healthy fats, omega-3s, and low toxicity, fish is a great place to start.

Fresh or Dried Fruit is always great for breastfeeding mothers! Eat the rainbow every day for the proper nutrients, vitamins, and minerals to regain strength and share it with your baby.

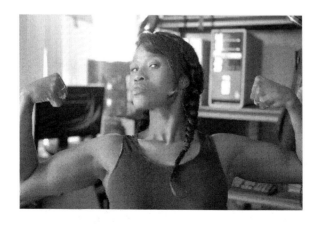

<u>Fresh Vegetables (with Hummus!)</u> is always great for breastfeeding mothers! Eat the rainbow every day for the proper nutrients, vitamins, and minerals to regain strength and share it with your baby.

<u>Leafy Greens</u> are high in magnesium for muscle and joint pain as well as fiber for healthy waste removal from your body (the last thing you want right now is to be constipated!). They also provide an incredible number of minerals for health in general, including vitamins A & C, calcium, and antioxidants.

<u>Lean Beef</u> boosts mama's energy with iron, protein, and vitamin B12, all of which are essential for her energy to be able to keep up with the baby.

<u>Low-Fat Dairy Products</u> such as milk, yogurt, or cheese provide vitamin D, calcium, protein, and more, all of which are essential for building strong bones and developing baby's immune system.

<u>Mushrooms</u> are thought to contain a lactogenic agent present in both barley and oats that help mothers produce milk for their newborns. The best mushrooms for the job are oyster, maitake, shimeji, shiitake, or reishi.

<u>Nuts</u> have so much going on that they should be part of the breastfeeding mother's daily diet. Nuts are high in zinc, calcium, iron, and vitamins K & B. They're also lactogenic, especially almonds, and they provide protein and fatty acids for mama in these times of need, too.

<u>Oranges</u> give a great energy boost through their vitamin C content.

Red & Orange Root Veggies have been used for their lactogenic potential in many cultures around the world for generations. In particular, carrots and yams are favored when it comes to using food to increase breastfeeding capacity.

Seeds (esp. Chia, Flax, & Hemp) in general are high in protein, calcium, iron, and zinc, but specifically, chia, flax, and hemp seeds are overloaded in omega-3 content. How perfect for a breastfeeding mom!

Starchy Foods (i.e. bread, potatoes, pasta, rice) provide an excellent source of energy for breastfeeding mothers. If you're intermittently fasting, be sure to include lots of these (balanced with healthy fats!) in your diet.

Turmeric, Fennel, Fenugreek, & Ashwagandha are all incredibly healing herbs that should be used in the cooking of all breastfeeding mothers. The first three are lactogenic, helping breastfeeding mothers produce milk, while the final one is a reproductive, glandular, immune, and neurological booster. It relieves stress, fights disease, and increases the quality of life for everyone who uses it.

Whole Wheat and Grains such as barley and oats are packed with lactogenic potential. They are essential for the breastfeeding mother's diet, especially if she's intermittently fasting.

5 IF recipes for Breastfeeding women

Strawberry Lactation Smoothie

This smoothie is the perfect snack or treat for a breastfeeding mom. It's packed with oats, berries, and other necessities to keep that milk coming without hesitation for baby.

This recipe needs less than five minutes of prep and less than five minutes of assembly. It will make one helping.

- Fat – 8.3 g
- Protein – 15.2 g
- Net Carbs – 72.6 g
- Calories – 411

What to Use:

- Milk or Unsweetened Alternative Milk (1 cup)
- Oats (0.5 cup)
- Banana (1)
- Strawberries (0.75 cup, frozen)
- Vanilla Extract (0.5 teaspoon)
- Agave Nectar (2 teaspoons)

What to Do:

- In a capable blender, combine all ingredients until perfectly smooth. Serve in a tall glass or split between two and enjoy

Easy Lactation-Aid Oatmeal

For a breastfeeding mom, morning breakfasts might be the one thing you just can't skip, and when you're craving that morning pick-me-up, there's nothing as easy as oatmeal. With some conscious meal prep, you'll have your breakfasts (or morning snacks) ready in wait with lactation aid provided through their ingredient lists.

This recipe needs about five minutes of prep and 5-10 minutes of cooking. It will make 2 helpings.

- Fat – 6.6 g
- Protein – 32.1 g
- Net Carbs – 45.9 g
- Calories – 365

What to Use:

- Oats (0.5 cup)
- Ground Flax Seed (2 teaspoons)
- Brewer's Yeast (0.5 teaspoon)
- Salt (to taste)
- Cinnamon (0.5 teaspoon)
- Water (1 cup)
- Milk or Alternative Milk (0-4 tablespoons, as desired)
- Honey or Agave Nectar (1-2 teaspoons, as desired)
- Additional toppings:
  - Dried or fresh fruit
  - Nuts
  - Seeds
  - Pre-made granola

What to Do:

- Start with a microwave-safe bowl (or heat-safe ceramic bowl), and combine the oats, flax seed, salt, cinnamon, and any additional toppings aside from fresh fruit.
- If you're using the microwave, next add in the brewer's yeast and water. Stir and microwave on high for 3 minutes. Stir when finished and let cool slightly. Add in milk, sweetener, and any additional fresh fruit as desired, and serve.
- If you're using the stovetop, boil 1.5 cups of water instead of just one cup. Once it has boiled, stir the water into your bowl with the dry ingredients. Stir in the yeast as well. Cover and let sit for 5 minutes. Uncover, add milk and sweetener, put on any fresh fruits, and serve.

Nursing Mom's Go-To Banana Bread

Packed with helpful lactation spices, this banana bread will help any nursing mom be able to balance better intermittent fasting and the task at hand with feeding her baby. It's a delicious recipe, to boot!

This recipe needs 20 minutes of prep and about an hour and a half of baking. It will make 8 helpings.

- Fat – 20.3 g
- Protein – 15.7 g
- Net Carbs – 63.7 g
- Calories – 488

What to Use:

- Ground Flax Seed (2 tablespoons)
- Water (4 tablespoons)
- Flour (1.75 cups)
- Oats (1.25 cups)
- Baking Soda (1 teaspoon)
- Salt (0.5 teaspoon)
- Brewer's Yeast (4 tablespoons)
- Ground Fenugreek (1 teaspoon)
- Cinnamon (0.5 teaspoon)
- Butter (0.5 cup, softened)
- Eggs (3, at room temperature)
- Agave (0.75 cup)
  - or Sugar (1 cup)
- Milk (2 tablespoons)
- Bananas (3 medium-sized or 2 large-sized, mashed)
- Vanilla Extract (1 teaspoon)
- Pecans (0.5 cup, chopped)

- or Walnuts (0.5 cup, chopped)
- or both! (0.25 cup of each, chopped)

What to Do:

- Start by preheating the oven. Turn it to 350 degrees and grab a 10-inch pan for a bread loaf. Grease the pan and set it aside
- Separately, mix together in a small-sized bowl the first two ingredients. Set that aside as well.
- In a medium-sized bowl, combine all the dry ingredients. Save the nuts for later though.
- In a larger bowl, use a handheld mixer to blend the butter, sugar or agave, eggs, milk, and mashed banana. Add flax goo and vanilla and blend until smooth.
- Set the handheld mixer aside and use a spatula to stir in one-third of the dry mixture at a time. Mix until just combined then add nuts.
- Pour mixture into loaf pan and bake. After 55-60 minutes, remove the bread and set it to cool. Serve hot or chilled!

Chicken & Barley Soup for Mom

This delicious soup will bring you great comfort and joy on a long day with the baby, and it's not even complicated to make! The best part is that it provides a great serving of protein, and for breastfeeding moms, it's productive because it relies on the healthy grain barley, which is a powerful lactation aid and hydrator.

This recipe needs 15 minutes of prep and about an hour of cooking. It will make 4 helpings.

- Fat – 6 g
- Protein – 31 g
- Net Carbs – 56 g
- Calories – 383

What to Use:

- Olive Oil (1 tablespoon)
- Onion (1 medium-sized, chopped)
- Button Mushrooms (1 pound, sliced)
- Carrots (2 medium-sized, peeled & diced)
- Baby Potatoes (1 pound, cut into inch piece)
- Garlic (3 cloves, minced)
- Vegetable Broth (4 cups)
- Water (1 cup)
- Pearl Barley (0.5 cup, rinsed with cold water)
- Chicken Breasts (2 deskinned & deboned, cubed)
- Peas (1 cup, frozen)

What to Do:

- Take a large-sized pot and set it on the stovetop on medium heat. Heat up the oil and add your onion. Cook about 5 minutes before adding your button mushrooms, carrots, potatoes, and minced garlic.
- Cook 5 minutes longer. Add liquids and barley grain.
- Bring soup to a boil, then reduce heat to low and simmer.
- Cover the soup and simmer 25-30 minutes.
- Stir in chicken and peas at this point and cook until both are done to your liking. The soup should be ready to serve about 10 minutes past this point.

Fish with Simple Beans & Greens

With a side of tasty beans and healthy greens, this fish filet will be the perfect meal for when you decide to breakfast. This recipe's reliance on nutrient-dense beans, leafy greens, and fishy omega-3s will help you absorb those nutrients so necessary to produce breastmilk for the little one.

This recipe needs 15 minutes of prep and 10 minutes of cooking. It will make 2 helpings.

- Fat – 27 g
- Protein – 45 g
- Net Carbs – 28 g
- Calories – 410

What to Use:

- Olive Oil (for sautéing: 1+ tablespoon, mild flavor)
- Chorizo (0.5 pound)
- Onion (1 medium-sized, chopped finely)
- Spinach (0.5 pound)
- Fish of choice (2 portions in filets):
  - Hake
  - Salmon
  - Tuna
  - Catfish
  - etc.
- Smoked Paprika (0.5 teaspoon)
- Red Chili (1 small-sized, deseeded & minced)
- Cannellini Beans (1 – 15 ounce can, drained & rinsed)
- Lemon Juice (2 tablespoons)
- Extra Virgin Olive Oil (1 tablespoon)

What to Do:

- Before you do anything else, put a kettle or pot of about 4 cups of water on to boil. You'll use this to make your spinach wilted later on.
- Now, turn the oven to high broil and, separately, heat up a frying pan on the stovetop with high heat. Add about a teaspoon of oil and place your chorizo into that heat. Stir quickly and add onion. Stir-fry for about 7 minutes until both the meat and onions are cooked completely. Remove from heat momentarily.
- Use that water to wilt your spinach. Place the half-pound of spinach in a strainer and pour that water over top. Set the spinach aside to drain.
- Take a baking sheet lined with aluminum foil to use for your fish. On the tray, pour a little of the oil and then your fish. Season the filets with paprika and a bit more of that oil.
- Take the frying pan back up to high heat with the sausages still there and the onions. Add the red chili and fry a moment longer.
- Then, pour on the beans, the wilted spinach greens, your extra virgin olive oil, and your lemon juice. Turn heat to low and allow to become warm. Season as needed.
- Take your fish and put it into the oven on broil. After five minutes, check the fish. If you need to turn it or adjust it on the tray, do so and broil 5-10 minutes longer, accordingly.
- Serve fish on top of beans and greens mixture and enjoy.

Chapter 9: Intermittent Fasting for the Woman with PCOS

Another subset of women that should be cautious when approaching intermittent fasting is those who struggle with PCOS. This acronym stands for a hormonal disorder called Polycystic Ovary Syndrome that causes the woman's reproductive system to dysfunction in certain ways that lead to pain, weight gain, missed periods, and hormonal imbalances of a variety of kinds.

While some people believe women with PCOS shouldn't overly stress their systems with something like intermittent fasting, others think that IF is exactly what these ladies need. In this chapter, we'll go over the details of PCOS as well as how intermittent fasting can actually help. Furthermore, we'll approach dietary tips, treatments, and exercises for women with this condition, and we'll end with the best IF-inspired ways for these women to lose weight.

By the end of this chapter, you should have a hunch whether or not you have PCOS, and if you already know that you have it, you should feel confident about whether or not intermittent fasting can help you. Regardless of what path you choose, the final three sections of this chapter should provide you with somewhat of a cheat-sheet to interact with the world on a more health-oriented level, whether through food, treatment, exercise, or weight loss.

What Is PCOS?

For women with PCOS, life can be miserable. Periods can be unpredictable, and these women's bodies can become almost like foreign worlds, what with all the hormones going haywire. Essentially, PCOS is a hormonal imbalance that affects the reproductive health and metabolism of those who live out the condition. This imbalance of reproductive hormones causes issues for these women's ovaries, causing them to have trouble releasing eggs as they should.

Although the name of the disorder speaks of cysts, many women do not develop cysts on their ovaries with this condition. Instead, all women with PCOS develop pools of excess fluids in their ovaries, they produce a surplus of androgens (commonly known as "male hormones"), they're all less responsive to insulin, and they all experience a relative lack of progesterone (which contributes more to those irregular periods).

The overall symptoms of PCOS are extra hair growth or early balding (caused by that androgen!), acne, headaches, mood swings, fatigue, weight gain, insomnia or light sleep, pelvic pain, and even infertility. Therefore, this disorder can make women extra cranky, heavy, sleepy, sad, and bald. It's not a fun fight! When it comes to PCOS, however, there are a couple of things you can try, and one of them is – you guessed it! – intermittent fasting.

How IF Helps with PCOS

As we learned in chapter 7, intermittent fasting can be helpful for certain women who experience constant stress, due to the abilities that IF grants your cells for regeneration alongside the effects of aging and disease. Therefore, that same effect for stressed-out people whereby intermittent fasting fends off internal inflammation and oxidative stress is also helpful for women struggling with PCOS! With less of this cellular stress, women with PCOS will likely find their overall health better and their struggle with their chronic disease all that much easier.

Intermittent fasting is also helpful for women who have extra bloat or just can't seem to lose weight due to their circumstances with PCOS. Limiting your caloric intake with intermittent fasting will surely give your metabolism the boost it needs, especially since your ability to regulate insulin in your body is affected through PCOS. For women like you, intermittent fasting will purposefully decrease insulin levels and increase human growth hormones, boosting your metabolism with a natural jolt of inspiration.

IF additionally works to fight depression, as we learned in chapter 7, which will make the situation for women with PCOS all the easier. Furthermore, the jolt to your system caused by IF triggers your cells to start repairing and removing waste while it encourages your blood levels of human growth hormone to increase. Ultimately, the effects associated are that you get fitter and feel better.

Best Foods & Diets for PCOS

Whether or not you decide to attempt intermittent fasting with PCOS, however, please make sure to speak with your doctor first. And if you *do* decide to combine the two, make sure you seek the most healthful, nutrition-dense foods you can for when you breakfast. The biggest concern for women with PCOS trying IF is that they're simply worried about losing weight when their bodies are going through something much more complex than just weight gain. By ensuring your food choices are healthy and supportive, you will work to heal yourself as a whole rather than just *one* side-effect of PCOS. Some healthful foods that go well with the condition and side-effects of PCOS are as follows.

- Meats, Fish, & Eggs
- Cold Water Fish (esp. Salmon & Sardines)
- Healthy Fats
- Probiotics (both in drinks & foods)
- Non-Starchy Vegetables
- Fruit (with restriction – see below)
- Carbohydrates (with restriction)
- Whole Foods (generally)
- Natural, Unprocessed Foods
- High-Fiber Foods
- Leafy Greens
- Dark Red & Blue Fruits (esp. Blueberries, Blackberries, Cherries, & Red Grapes)
- Beans & Legumes
- Nuts
- Spices (esp. Turmeric & Cinnamon)
- Dark Chocolate (with restriction)
- Cruciferous Vegetables
- Squash (of all types)
- Anti-Inflammation Foods (i.e. Tomatoes, Kale, Spinach, Almonds, Walnuts, Olive Oil, Blueberries, Fatty Fish, Etc.)
- Green (& other flavors of) Tea

You may decide that intermittent fasting isn't right for you, given your condition, after all. In this case, you can still work to lose that pesky weight! You just might have to switch gears back to *what's* being eaten, rather than *when* it's consumed. You'll want to make sure that you don't restrict too much from your diet, so (for example) a completely raw, plant-based diet *might* take too much from you when you still need a lot of what that diet could never provide. Be careful, too, about fad diets that you haven't researched into for yourself (such as the lectin-free and keto diets). Some diets that work well for people with PCOS are as follows.

Vegan Diet (or restricted-dairy Vegetarian Diet): If you're able to cut out meat in your diet (and interested in doing so), you might find that the Vegan Diet provides restriction of dairy in ways that help with your condition. However, you'll have to steer clear of bingeing on gluten and soy in substitution, for those are not friendly to people with PCOS! You could also try a Dairy-Restricted Vegetarian diet. There are certainly options to play around with until things feel right (or at least better) inside.

Dairy-Restricted Diet: A Dairy-Restricted Diet might be the best middle ground for someone in your shoes. You might not be interested in cutting meat out of your diet, but knowing that dairy is unhelpful, just focus on that. Cut out dairy completely or limit your intake to only once a day. The less you consume, the better, and it can happen one step at a time.

Gluten-Restricted Diet: Gluten adds to inflammation in the body, which makes things difficult for women with PCOS who already have a lot of inflammation in their bodies. What makes matters worse is that the more inflammation we have, the more insulin-resistant we become (bad!), and the more testosterone exists in our bodies (bad for you, PCOS lady!). The problem gets a little tougher because many gluten-free alternatives are super-refined, meaning that they're not good for your insulin levels either. So the trick will be to avoid or restrict gluten without going to gluten-free alternatives. That's going to be interesting...

No-GMO Diet: Highly modified food products like gluten and corn tend to aggravate conditions for women with PCOS, but another one that's less noticed is soy. Soy is hugely modified compared to its original existence as a seed and plant, but soy also makes hormonal issues for women with PCOS all the worse. Soy makes ovulation even more delayed for women, whether or not they have PCOS, so it really should be avoided along with other genetically-modified foods.

Sugar-Restricted Diet: Sugar, even in fruit, can be problematic for people with PCOS. Processed and refined sugar, in particular, is detrimental for women with PCOS who hope to get pregnant someday because they decrease the quality of your eggs, increase rates of miscarriage, and reduce your sex drive as well. Even the fructose in fruits can make your insulin production wonky and contribute to weight gain if you overly rely on fruits in your diet. Try to cut out processed sugars but limit that fresh fruit consumption, too. Your situation will certainly be made better.

Best Treatments & Exercises for PCOS

Whether you want to combine PCOS with intermittent fasting or not, there are a few other treatments and exercises to consider to mitigate the effects of your condition. After trying out a few of these, if things still haven't gotten better, maybe a more drastic measure such as intermittent fasting will help you more. It's hard to say for sure at this moment, but as always, move forward with your doctor's approval to ensure your path to health is the best one for the situation.

As far as treatments go, there are a few directions you can go. There are (1) medicinal treatments, (2) alleviation of symptom treatments, and (3) lifestyle treatments. In terms of medicinal treatments, you could try using a birth control method (i.e. the pill, the patch, the shot, an IUD, or the vaginal ring) that works primarily on hormones. This will help regulate your period, lower cancer risk, and help with the acne and hair issues. You could also try medicines that block androgens in your body to get rid of that acne and hair loss. These pills are often problematic if you want to become pregnant in the future, though. Additionally, you could try Metformin (used to treat type 2 diabetes, but helps with PCOS symptoms too); Provera (regulates menses through providing progesterone); Clomiphene/Clomid, Letrozole/Femara, or Gonadotropins (medications that help increase and regulate ovulation); Eflornithine or Electrolysis (to help with slowing facial hair growth, if necessary); or Progestin therapy (protects against cancer and regulates periods, but won't help with androgen). Many of these medical treatments are treatments that tie into symptom-alleviation as well.

The third option is lifestyle treatments, whereby bigger decisions and life changes are meant to help the individual heal and cope with their disorder. In this case, fasting, IF, or dieting are great additions along with exercise. If and when you decide to incorporate exercise into your lifestyle (to help heal or otherwise), you can make sure your workouts include one or more of these five tactics so that you're getting the most out of the experience (in ways that benefit your condition, too).

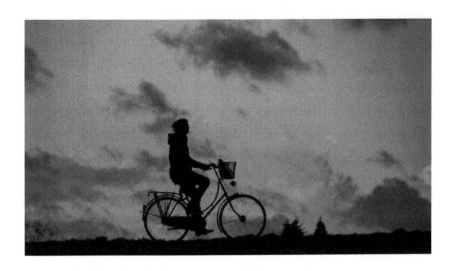

First, go for some cardio. Cardio training has abilities to increase mood, stabilize fertility, and help with your insulin resistance issue. Whether it's walking, jogging, cycling, swimming, or otherwise, even just 30 minutes a day of cardio works wonders on your weight while helping with other side-effects of PCOS. If you do nothing else, incorporate cardio into your daily routine, and you'll already be feeling better in no time.

Second, try strength training! Equally helpful for your insulin resistance issue, strength training like cardio improves insulin function in the body while boosting metabolism and contributing to good moods.

Third, if you've never heard of the pelvic floor, you're in for a "treat"! You can always use pelvic floor strengthening to lessen that pelvic pain and tension that you might feel on a daily basis. You don't even need to go to the gym to do this. All you have to do is squeeze your butt-cheeks together. You'll feel that, nearer to your vulva, you have another squeezing occurring, too. See if you can isolate that sensation. As you get better at doing exactly that, you'll become able to squeeze for five breaths and release.

The longer you can complete these repetitions of squeezing and releasing, the stronger your pelvic floor will be! There are also tools you can find in certain stores and online that are oriented towards pelvic floor strengthening when you get to that point.

Fourth, work on that core strength! Core strength not only makes your body stronger, but it also helps increase senses of well-being and personal power. When your core is strong, you have a much easier time knowing what you want, speaking out about it, and saying "no" when you need to. Just like pelvic floor strengthening, working on core strength will be hugely beneficial when/if you decide to become pregnant.

Fifth, if you're feeling up to it, try HIIT. High-Intensity Interval Training can help you lose 5-10% of your original weight, which is always going to help mitigate PCOS symptoms. The more weight you lose, the less androgen and testosterone are stocked up in your body, and the better insulin resistance you develop.

Best (IF) Tips on How to Lose Weight for PCOS

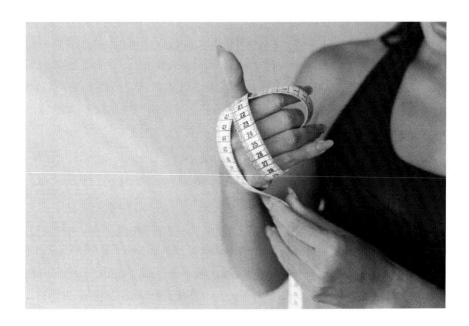

Overall, losing weight with PCOS is a great goal. Losing weight can help your symptoms become lessened in many ways. It can help your body remember how to regulate insulin; it can help your hormones go back to normal levels; it can help provide daily activity; it can make your body healthier and stronger; and if you want to get pregnant despite your condition, losing weight is an essential step to recover your fertility. A few tips to lose weight through intermittent fasting and otherwise, are listed below.

<u>Try out crescendo method!</u> If you do decide to explicitly incorporate intermittent fasting into your routine as someone with PCOS, go with crescendo method. Start with just one or two days on a 14:14 fast, and then if the first week feels good on all

levels, you might consider trying those one or two days on 16:8 instead, or switching to three days at 14:14. The crescendo method is built to be flexible, so try it out and then see if your body wants (and allows) you to stick with it.

Delay your breakfast! You can still try to get that 12-hour, 14-hour, or even 16-hour fast in the right at the beginning of your day by just waiting a little longer for breakfast.

Eat dinner earlier! If you really want to incorporate IF into your PCOS life, try eating dinner earlier to begin your fast each night. You'll easily be able to get 12 or 14 of fast in daily with that adjustment.

Cut out those snacks! You might not be able to try fasting windows each day, and it could be the case that you do try them, and it doesn't make anything better. Instead, try cutting down on your daily snack intake! That simple dietary switch can help enact IF goals in your life as well as its side-effects.

Eat healthier meals! Instead of fasting or exercising intensely, you could always switch to eating healthier meals when you decide it's time to eat. There are some women with PCOS who only have to make this slight adjustment to see the weight loss goals they desire.

Reconsider serving sizes! This point goes hand-in-hand with the one before it. If you redesign your meals to be healthier, whether in content or serving size, you may be able to see your weight loss goals actualized without intermittent fasting whatsoever.

Mesh exercise with dietary change! Since you might decide *not* to engage with intermittent fasting, given your condition, just be reminded that you can always combine exercise routine and dietary change to achieve the same effects. While women who intermittently fast are often discouraged from incorporating both intense exercise *and* dietary change into their routine while practicing IF, you don't have to worry about that goal-clash as much.

Chapter 10: Intermittent Fasting for the Mature or Menopausal Woman

While the greatest concerns about intermittent fasting's effects on women often center on potential problems with reproduction and fertility, some women simply don't have to worry about that anymore. For mature and menopausal women, intermittent fasting poses a different instance and option entirely.

This chapter will be dedicated to the experiences of these women. It will discuss what happens when women age, how their needs change, and how nutrition is affected. Furthermore, it will discuss how intermittent fasting affects both mature and menopausal women before giving suggestions of how to approach IF for each type of woman.

Next, we will walk through some anti-aging foods, tips, and exercises to lose that weight, and then we'll end with the best intermittent fasting method for you at this time. By the time this chapter ends, you should feel confident (as a mature or menopausal woman) that you can approach intermittent fasting safely and productively, and you should have a solid plan in mind regarding how you'll go about that when you're ready.

Differences Between the Young vs. Older Woman

At the most basic level, it must be said that there are detailed bodily differences between young women and older women. Many of these bodily differences become obvious with the outward, physical effects of aging, but a lot of them also happen on the inside, away from what our eyes can see.

When women age, enter and exit menopause, and become fully mature, their bodies change, reflecting different nutritional needs for the next 30+ years. During menopause, in particular, certain foods help with the urges, hot flashes, and more, but the period of intense transition is more of a gateway into a completely altered future (mentally, bodily, nutritionally, and more).

Women of this age experience slowed metabolism (to their great frustrations) as well as lowered hormone production. For weight and mood, therefore, menopause and maturation are equal disasters. Your body will go completely "out of whack," compared to how it used to function. You'll likely put on weight despite the dietary choices you make, and you may feel there's no relief in sight. Don't be fooled, however! Things may have changed for you, but they won't be stagnant changes.

Essentially, women at the stage of menopause and beyond need to absorb less energy overall from their food, yet they need more protein to deal with the effects of aging. Vitamins B12 & D, calcium, and zinc will need to be boosted, while iron becomes less important for the aging female body. Vitamins C, E, A, & beta-carotene need to be increased too in order to fight off cancer, infection, disease, and more.

As the woman ages and matures even further, more things will change; mainly, she cannot bypass taking these important supplements any longer. In older and more mature women, the body's abilities to recognize hunger and thirst become muted, and dehydration poses a greater threat. Fewer calories are required for the older and more mature woman too, but she still needs to get as many nutrients as (if not more than!) the young woman does.

It seems that a younger woman can eat (relatively) what she wants and not worry about taking vitamins or supplements, but it is undeniable that the older woman will need this nutritional help to *ensure* longevity. Basically, health needs become more pressing for women at this age, as their bodies are less flexible and resistant to problems that may arise.

How IF Affects Women at This Age & How to Approach It

Because health, diet, reproductivity, and nutritional needs are all altered for mature and menopausal women, their relationships with intermittent fasting can be very different from young women's. For instance, while young women ought to be careful about how intermittent fasting can affect their fertility levels, older women can practice intermittent fasting freely without these concerns. Therefore, more mature women can apply the weight-loss techniques of intermittent fasting to their lives (and waistlines) without worry of what negative side-effects might arise in the future.

For menopausal women, however, the situation is a little bit different than it is for fully mature women. People going through menopause have to deal with daily hormone fluctuations that cause hot and cold flashes, sleeplessness, anxiety, irregular periods, and more. At the beginning of this process, intermittent fasting *will not* necessarily help, and it could even make your situation more stressful.

For women in this situation who are actively going through menopause, you must remember that your body is extremely sensitive to changes right now. If you do find that intermittent fasting helps and that short periods of fast are effective, you *must* also make sure to increase the intensity of your fast as gradually as possible so your body can adjust without creating horrible hormonal repercussions for yourself and everyone around you.

For the fully mature woman, intermittent fasting will not make you as cranky, moody, irregular in the period, or otherwise because those hormones won't be affecting you at all anymore, or at least, hardly at all. Your dietary and eating schedule choices become more liberated from the effects they used to have on your hormonal health as the years go by. Therefore, if you're seeking weight loss, better energy, a physiological jolt back to health, or what have you, try out IF without concern and see what happens. For these types of women, intermittent fasting is set to provide hope through eased depression, the lessened likelihood of cancer (or its recurrence), promised weight loss, and more.

Anti-Aging Foods

Avocado is high in omega-3s, which help your immune system as well as your body as a whole fight inflammation.

Beans & Lentils are great sources of protein and fiber, particularly for older women.

Blueberries are high in vitamin C and antioxidants that help protect the skin from pollutants, sun exposure, aging stress, and more.

Broccoli, Cauliflower, & Brussel Sprouts are all relatively high in lutein which keeps your brain healthy and sharp!

<u>Carrots</u> are also rich in vitamin A as well as beta-carotene which helps your vision later in life.

<u>Cilantro</u> might taste like soap to some, but it helps remove metals from your body that shouldn't be there. It's a great detoxifier for women of any age.

<u>Cooked Tomatoes</u> have a powerful antioxidant present that helps the skin heal from the damage of any kind.

<u>Dark Chocolate</u> is packed with flavanols (which aid in the appearance of the skin and protect against the damage of the sun).

<u>Edamame</u> aids in bone health, cardiovascular healing, and ease into lowered estrogen levels with menopause.

<u>Fortified Plant-Based Milk</u> is a great non-dairy alternative to the "healing" animal milk you may know and love. They provide bone-supportive minerals and nutrients like calcium and vitamin D (as long as they're fortified!) without adding in the problematic nature of dairy to your healthy drink.

<u>Ghee</u> is a special form of clarified butter that is packed with healthy fats for skin health and detoxification.

<u>Green Tea</u> de-stresses the body and mind and blocks DNA from damage in many forms.

<u>Manuka Honey</u> is a special type of honey that's a powerful natural remedy for immune boost and skin health.

<u>Mushrooms</u> are high in vitamin D, which is so important for women of all ages.

Nuts are great at lowering cholesterol and fighting inflammation. They're also packed with fiber, protein, and micronutrients.

Oatmeal provides carbohydrates that encourage the release of serotonin, which keeps you feeling good.

Olives provide polyphenols and other essential phytonutrients that keep your DNA protected and your skin and body feeling and looking young.

Oranges, Lemons, & Limes, when juiced, provide the greatest source of healthy vitamin C you can imagine.

Papaya has many antioxidants, vitamins, and minerals that keep the skin elastic with fewer wrinkle lines.

Pineapples help maintain skin health, elasticity, and strength as you age.

Pomegranate Seeds are also high in antioxidants, and they're great at fighting free radical molecules that encourage the effects of aging on the body.

Red & Orange Bell Peppers have antioxidants and high vitamin C to help the skin retain its healthy shine while protecting it against pollutants and toxins.

Red Wine, when drunk in moderation, is a powerful tool to keep your heart healthy, lower cholesterol, and maintain muscle mass.

Saffron has anti-tumor, antioxidant, and other highly nutritious effects for the body.

Sesame Seeds will help you feel good through their high levels of calcium, magnesium, fiber, phosphorous, and iron.

Spinach & Other Leafy Greens work to protect the skin from sun damage while providing beta-carotene and lutein to solidify that effect.

Sweet Potato has more vitamin A than regular potatoes, which keeps your skin fresh and young-looking without lines and wrinkles.

Turmeric is great for the skin and for keeping the organs working in tip-top shape. The pigment curcumin also helps to heal DNA and prevent degenerative diseases.

Watercress is a happily hydrating green that's high in phosphorous, manganese, calcium, potassium, vitamins A, C, K, B1, and B2.

Watermelon works like a natural sun blocker when eaten and provides a great source of water to keep you hydrated.

Yogurt helps your cells stay young and is often probiotic, which is great for healthy gut flora and mood stabilization.

Tips & Exercises to Lose Belly Fat & Kickstart Your Metabolism

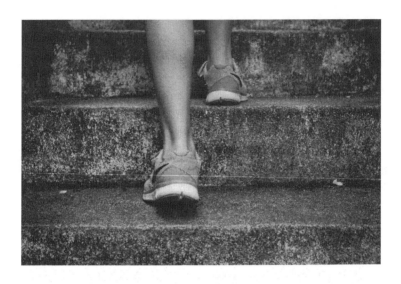

If you're eager to lose that belly fat associated with menopause and give your metabolism a kick-start to the face, you're definitely in the right place! Whether or not you choose to incorporate intermittent fasting into your life, there are still several things you can do to make sure these goals are achieved exactly as you want them to be.

The two biggest tips for losing this belly fat are (1) to switch your diet to something that triggers fat loss and fat burning and (2) to start a new exercise regimen. While the intermittent fasting plan is not technically a diet, this switch in when you eat might be exactly what you need. If not, however, a few true diets you can try are The Low-Carb Diet, whereby you reduce the number of carbs you take in each day; The Mediterranean Diet, which is essentially vegetarian and plant-based aside from the occasional red meat and a few other switches; the Vegetarian Diet, which is shown to be particularly effective at helping overweight post-menopausal women lose the fat they desire; and then the more intense Vegan Diet, which boasts the same effects as The Vegetarian Diet, just with more conclusive, less age-restrictive results.

Altering your diet is just one step, however. You also have to be exercising enough to burn the fat that's present. Given your age, your ability, and any other circumstances, you'll want to find a mode of exercise that's not too demanding or stressful. Somethings that could work for you are Resistance Training with low weights and bands, Aerobic Cardio, Aerobic Exercise otherwise, and Low-Demand Strength Training. Daily walks are also incredibly helpful for women in your situation to be able to reach their weight loss goals. If you can manage it, a combination of Aerobic and Resistance Exercises is ideal.

Best (IF) Methods for Health & Weight Loss at This Age

For the menopausal woman, the best method to start with would be something low-stress and gradual. The crescendo method sure is gradual, but it may be a little too intense for the menopausal woman to use as a beginner. If you do start with a crescendo, try two days a week at 12:12 or 14:10 at the toughest. If that feels okay, that's great, but you still should probably not make things any more forceful.

Instead of trying the crescendo method whatsoever, I would suggest the woman in this situation try spontaneous skip method first to see how things feel. If she's too moody, frustrated, hot-flashy, and upset with just this adjustment, I suggest she wait a few months until trying intermittent fasting again. If this phase goes well, she can up the ante and try 12:12 method, then 14:10 and 16:8 when she's ready. I doubt the menopausal woman would want to venture beyond these first four starting methods, however, given the bodily situation she's working through.

On the flip side, for the fully mature, post-menopausal woman, any method would be fine to start with. If the woman is unsure about starting off with day-by-day fierceness in her IF experience, she can try working with 12:12 method, working up to 14:10 method, and 16:8 if things feel okay. Even crescendo method would work well for the woman in this situation because she could determine how strict the "day-by-day" aspect was and make the schedule work in her favor. Any woman in this case likely won't *want* to start with the most rigorous intermittent fast, so these hourly-based ones offer a smoother initial transition.

If the woman in this situation has worked with intermittent fasting before, she is free to choose whichever method she prefers. If the mature woman has established a career for herself later in life and lives full days with evenings free, she is invited to try the warrior method. As long as she's taking supplements and drinking enough liquids, even this strenuous, appropriately-named diet can even be tackled by the oldest of women among us!

Chapter 11: Autophagy & Intermittent Fasting for Women

Would you believe me if I said that the biggest benefit of intermittent fasting wasn't weighted loss? Would you believe me if I said it wasn't the ability to have a clearer mind either? It's not about weight loss, mental capacity, or anything else as much as it is about what's called Autophagy.

This chapter is all about Autophagy; what it does in the body, what it means for health, and how it interacts with (and is triggered by) intermittent fasting. We'll start with the technical details before going into what this all means for women's health as a whole, and then by the end of the chapter, we'll touch on how Autophagy explicitly relates to intermittent fasting and what it can do for you.

By the time this chapter is through, you should feel affirmed in your belief that intermittent fasting both heals and rejuvenates the human body. At this point, and of course, due to the existence of Autophagy; this newfound, brilliant, and Nobel Prize-winning process, you should have no remaining doubts about what good intermittent fasting can do for you.

What Is Autophagy? What Is Protein Cycling?

Very simply, Autophagy is the relatively newfound ability that cells have, enabling them to recycle their parts that aren't working, to clear up the muck, to get rid of what's unhelpful, and to throw out their trash essentially. And what Autophagy gets rid of also are technically pathogenic microbes such as mold, fungus, bacteria, the virus that may be sitting in the cell that causes potential disorders, conditions, or diseases when they're allowed to stay in the cell.

Autophagy is an amazing physiological process, for its effects go as far as healing the brain, increasing and furthering anti-aging capacities, and significantly boosting immunity. It really goes to show that intermittent fasting enacts wide-spread healing on the body, rather than just helping it lose weight or look younger.

Protein Cycling is also related to Autophagy in that it helps your body and your cells work to recycle what isn't working through phases of protein consumption. Essentially, Protein Cycling is a process you can engage in to increase the anti-aging capacity of your intermittent fasting practice. What you do is alternate between times where you eat a lot of protein and times where you hardly eat any. When you're eating a lot of protein, you'll have high insulin levels and low glucagon (a hormone that works alongside yet opposite insulin to keep glucose levels in the blood at balance). But when you switch to low protein levels, your insulin levels will lower and glucagon levels will spike, meaning that (scientifically and physiologically) Autophagy is active and working in the body.

Autophagy, Protein Cycling, and Women's Health

When women decide to take command of their health, incredible things can happen. Whether you're older or younger, Autophagy as a process in the body is one of those incredible things, and it happens without you even thinking about it. However, you can also make choices that increase the occurrence of Autophagy, which only makes those incredible things in your body (your potential for self-guided healing, etc.) have a more profound effect.

For menopausal women, in particular, Autophagy creates a turnover of cells that helps the transition from young to mature. It helps in keeping these women's skin young, their limbs lose, their moods bright, and their transitions smooth overall. For women of all other ages, Autophagy gets rid of the gunk that keeps holding you back. It helps you move into new growth as well as the next stage of life with confidence. For women's health overall, Autophagy is utterly vital, and Protein Cycling only aids its occurrence and proper function.

How IF Affects People (concerning to Autophagy)

When paired with Protein Cycling, intermittent fasting can enact substantial and long-lasting healing for the body and the individual as a whole. Intermittent fasting, of course, effects people like a jolt to their systems, helping things be more productive and efficient. Also, IF causes Autophagy in the body, encouraging the cells to get rid of their "trash" and be healthier overall. When paired with Protein Cycling, though, intermittent fasting becomes almost like a real-world video game "cheat," but for weight loss, mental prowess, anti-aging abilities, and general well-being.

With Autophagy happening in the body, which only happens during low protein-intake or fasting states, your organs, your skin, your cells, your brain, your limbs, and more get a jolt of self-cleansing potential, and that possibility is incredible. You can take full advantage of that opportunity in yourself by engaging in conscious fasting in whatever intermittent plan works best for you.

As always, you may have to work through several methods to find the right one. But as long as you're Protein Cycling (an action inherent to intermittent fasting) in any regard, you'll ignite Autophagy and by doing so, you'll unintentionally save your own life again and again. What more could you ask for?

Chapter 12: 12 Useful Recipes for Weight Loss with Intermittent Fasting

If you're in need of a few recipes to get yourself in gear regarding health and whole foods during the transitions of intermittent fasting, look no further! The following pages include 12 recipes, ranging from breakfast, lunch, and dinner to dessert and snacks in between. This chapter will provide details on which recipes do *what* for you, in healing terms, as well, so you should not only know what *meals* to make but also you will know what *the ingredients* are doing for you on the inside.

Breakfast Recipes

Yogurt with Berries & Chia Seeds

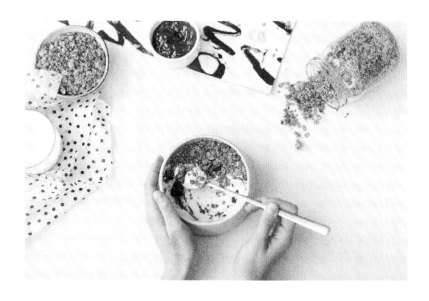

To have breakfast with ease for your body and mind, try this light, energy-inducing, probiotic, and antioxidizing starter. Add whatever you'd like for toppings!

This recipe needs 5-10 minutes of prep and requires no baking or cooking time. It will make two helpings.

- Fat – 11.2 g
- Protein – 15.7 g
- Net Carbs – 25.4 g
- Calories – 310

What to Use:

- Yogurt (1.5-2 cups)
- Berries of Choice (1 handful)
- Chia Seeds (1 tablespoon)
- Additional Toppings, as desired:
  - Berry Compote or Jam (1-2 tablespoons)
  - Oats or Granola (2-5 tablespoons)
  - Dried Fruits (as desired)
  - Nuts & Seeds (as desired)

What to Do:

- Simply pour your yogurt into a cup or bowl, sprinkle with chia seeds, add the fruit, and enjoy!
- If you desire extra toppings, add them as needed.

DIY Omelet for Your Needs

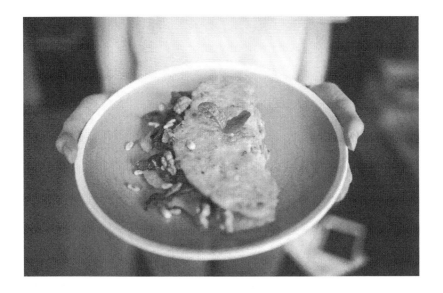

Eggs are so good for you, especially when you need meals that are easy and packed with protein! Omelets, in particular, are wonderful because the inside additions allow you to get creative and heal yourself all at once. Don't hold back with the inventiveness here!

This recipe needs 5-10 minutes of prep and about 5 minutes of cooking. It will make one helping.

- Fat – 24.4 g
- Protein – 18.6 g
- Net Carbs – 4.1 g
- Calories – 220

What to Use:

- Eggs (2-3, large-sized)
- Milk (0.25 cup)
- Salt & Pepper (to taste)

- Additions, as desired:
    o Vegetables, such as red or green pepper, greens, sprouts, etc.
    o Nuts & Seeds
    o Herbs, such as basil, thyme, rosemary, oregano, cilantro, etc.
    o Drizzles for Garnish, such as balsamic vinegar, olive oil, cheese, etc.

What to Do:

- Grab a small skillet and heat the stovetop to about medium heat. In the skillet, melt a tablespoon of butter or spray with cooking spray.
- In a small separate bowl, mix the eggs, milk, salt, and pepper with a fork or whisk until smooth. Pour into heated & greased pan.
- Cook omelet fully on the bottom then flip.
- Add fillings (heated or raw) & serve.

Lunch Recipes

Fish Tacos with Lemon Dill Slaw

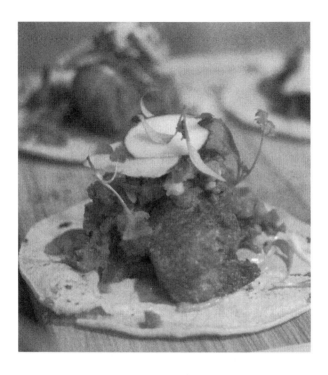

Fish is packed with omega-3s, so salmon is especially healthy for people working with intermittent fasting. Given the protein and the other nutrients in this recipe, you'll be coming back for more in no time.

This recipe needs 15-20 minutes of prep and 30 minutes of cooking. It will make 4 helpings of tacos.

- Fat – 30 g
- Protein – 31 g
- Net Carbs – 44 g
- Calories – 559

What to Use:

- For the Tacos
    - Salmon (4-4 ounce filets)
    - Ancho or Chili Powder (1 tablespoon)
    - Lime Juice (1 tablespoon)
    - Salt (0.25 teaspoon)
    - Pepper (0.25 teaspoon)
    - Tortillas (8-6 inch tortillas)
- For the Slaw
    - Red Cabbage (1 small-sized, shredded)
    - Green Cabbage (1 small-sized, shredded)
    - Lemon Juice (0.33 cup)
    - Dill (2 tablespoons, dried herb)
    - Salt & Pepper (to taste)
    - Mayonnaise (0.25 cup+, as needed)

What to Do:

- Turn on the stovetop to medium-high heat and spray a skillet with cooking spray (or melt a tablespoon of butter). Season your salmon filets and then add them to the skillet. Cook about 5 minutes on each side of filet until cooked through.
- Remove the salmon skin and then flake the "meat" into taco-sized chunks.
- Separately, mix the shredded cabbage and seasonings. Taste your slaw to ensure it's right for your desires.
- Warm the tortillas if desired, and add about 0.5 cup salmon, 0.25 cup slaw to each one to serve. Eat while hot

Late-Summer Salad

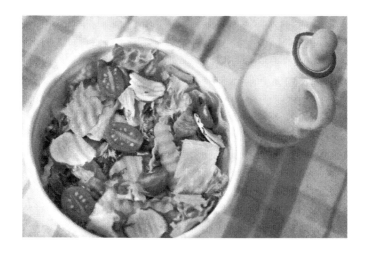

With all the cruciferous veggies in this salad, your body will be thanking you. Try this for a refreshing and mouthwatering healthy snack or a full meal, depending on your hunger level.

This recipe needs about 15 minutes of prep and requires no cooking or baking. It will make eight helpings.

- Fat – 9.5 g
- Protein – 8.7 g
- Net Carbs – 63.7 g
- Calories – 204

What to Use:

- Kale (1 pound, destemmed & chopped)
- Spring Mix (0.75 pound)
- Brussel Sprouts (10 sprouts, shredded)
- Cauliflower (1 medium-sized head, crumbled into "rice")
- Carrots (1 medium-sized, grated)
- Cherry Tomatoes (10-15, halved)

- Cranberries (0.33 cup, dried)
- Almonds (0.5 cup, sliced)
- Feta Cheese (0.66 cup, crumbled)
- Raspberry Vinaigrette:
  - Raspberries (2 cups, fresh or thawed from frozen)
  - Sugar (2 tablespoons)
  - Balsamic Vinegar (1.33 cups)
  - Olive Oil (0.5 cup)
  - Honey (2 tablespoons)
  - Salt (1 teaspoon)

What to Do:

- Prepare the dressing first of all by whisking together the berries and sugar first in a small bowl. Keep whisking until things become less gritty and juicier. Then, pour the mixture into a jar with a lid and add the remaining ingredients. Shake to combine. If you want your dressing smoother, put it through a blender before serving.
- Prepare the vegetables and greens for your salad and combine them into a large bowl when ready. Serve with cranberries, almonds, and feta as somewhat of a garnish.
- If needed, cook any type of meat for an additional protein-packed topping.

Tri-Color Potato & Black Bean Hash

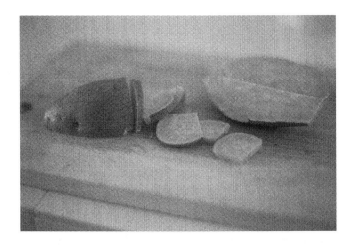

This snack is full of healthy carbohydrates and more, what with the colors, the complex starches, and the beans. It's delicious, and it's so, so good for you.

This recipe needs 5 minutes of prep and 15 minutes of cooking. It will make four helpings.

- Fat – 16.2 g
- Protein – 27.1 g
- Net Carbs – 102.1 g
- Calories – 641

What to Use:

- Olive Oil (4 tablespoons)
- Sweet Potato (1.5 cups, diced)
- Yukon Gold Potato (1.5 cups, diced)
- Purple Potato (1.5 cups, diced)
- Onion (1 small-sized, diced)
- Red Bell Pepper (1 large-sized, diced)

- Salt & Pepper (to taste)
- Paprika (0.5 teaspoon)
- Cumin (1 teaspoon)
- Spinach (2 cups, chopped)
- Black Beans (1-15 ounce can, drained & rinsed)

What to Do:

- With a large skillet, heat your tablespoons of oil on medium-high heat. When it's hot, add in the three colors of potatoes. Stir for 3-5 minutes then add the onion, salt, pepper, paprika, and cumin.
- Stir together and cook for about 10 minutes.
- Eventually, add the spinach and black beans, stir until heated through and everything is tender. Serve hot!

Snack Recipes

Homemade Trail Mix

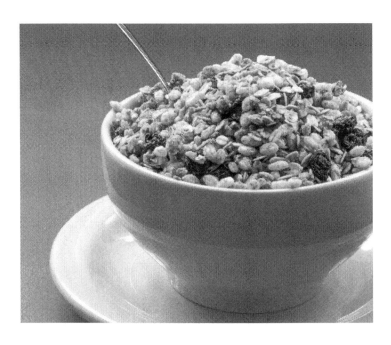

For that basic pick-me-up in the afternoon or morning, turn to your own, homemade trail mix. I promise, making it is much easier than it sounds!

This recipe needs 10 minutes of prep and 15 minutes of baking. It will make six helpings.

- Fat – 15.6 g
- Protein – 6.1 g
- Net Carbs – 75 g
- Calories – 460

What to Use:

- Rolled Oats (2 cups)
- Walnuts (0.25 cup)
- Almonds (0.25 cup)
- Pumpkin Seeds (2 tablespoons)
- Sunflower Seeds (2 tablespoons)
- Chia Seeds (2 teaspoons)
- Dried Cranberries (0.33 cup)
- Dried Mango (2 strips, chopped)
- Maple Syrup (3 tablespoons)
- Coconut Oil (2 tablespoons, melted)
- Vanilla Extract (0.5 teaspoon)
- Salt (1 large-sized pinch)

What to Do:

- Preheat the oven at 300 degrees and grab a large mixing bowl.
- Stir together all the ingredients in this large mixing bowl until it's all well-coated.
- With a large-sized, lined baking sheet, spread out your granola. Make a thin layer that's not too thick or piled up so that cooking happens as burn-free and effortlessly as possible.
- Toast for 5 minutes, stir, then toast for another 5 minutes.
- After 10 minutes and things are looking cooked but not burnt, take out the tray and cook your granola.
- This mixture can be stored for up to two weeks, but make sure it's in an air-tight container as storage and that it's completely cooled before transfer into this container! Eat alone as a snack or on yogurt with berries.

Homemade Grainy (Avocado) Toast

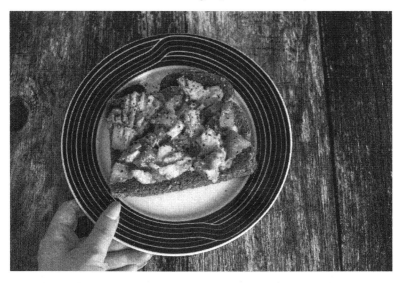

Bread doesn't have to be hard to make! Through this simple loaf recipe, you can have homemade bread and toast anytime. All you need is a little avocado on top to spruce things right up!

This recipe needs 2-5 hours of prep and about an hour of baking. It will make ten helpings.

- Fat – 0.1 g
- Protein – 2.6 g
- Net Carbs – 15 g
- Calories – 70

What to Use:

- Water (3 cups, lukewarm)
- Yeast (1.5 tablespoons)
- Salt (1.5 tablespoons)
- Whole Wheat Flour (6.5 cups)
- Cornmeal (for table dusting)

- Water (1 cup, boiling)
- Toppings, as desired:
  - Avocado (1, sliced)
  - Tomato (1 medium-sized, sliced or chopped)
  - Balsamic Vinegar (a sprinkle)
  - Garlic Spread (2 tablespoons)
  - Hummus & Olives (2 tablespoons & 0.25 cup, sliced)
  - Tapenade (2 tablespoons)
  - Butter & Jam (1 tablespoon, each)

What to Do:

- Start by preparing the dough. With three cups of lukewarm water at your side in a large bowl, mix the yeast and salt with the water. Make sure all the flour gets wet and then set the dough in the bottom of the bowl. Cover it with a lid that's not necessarily air-tight.
- Let the dough rise anywhere from 2-5 hours.
- When you're ready to bake, sprinkle some excess flour on the dough and then cut out a chunk about the size of a grapefruit. A serrated knife will help with this effort. Pull the dough lightly in your hands and then form something that has a rounded-off top and bumpy bottom part. Sprinkle with cornmeal and let rest for no longer than 45 minutes.
- *Repeat the previous step as many times as needed to process all the dough. Each ball will become a small loaf. You can cover and refrigerate this dough for up to two weeks*
- Preheat your oven to 450 degrees. Grab a baking stone and set it on the oven's middle rack so that it becomes hot. "Preheat" the baking stone in this way for about 20 minutes.

- Once the time is up, uncover your dough and dust it with flour. Take that serrated knife again and make three shallow slashes in the top of the loaf. Before placing this loaf in the oven, grab a shallow pan and set it in the bottom of the broiler.
- When you're ready, slide the dough onto your hot baking stone and pour a cup of boiling water into the pan to create steam and shut the oven immediately to trap that good baking steam!
- Check the loaf around 30 minutes, as it should be just about done. You want a well-browned loaf. Remove and cool before serving.
- Once the loaf is ready to cut, slice it and prepare a piece for toast. Use whatever toppings you desire!

Dinner Recipes

Salmon with Wild Rice & Greens

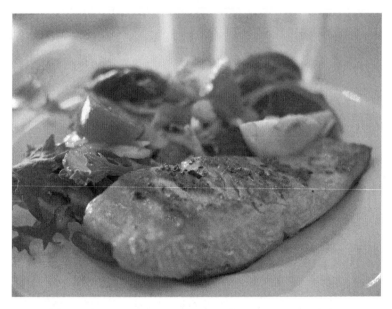

Another soon-to-be salmon favorite is coming your way! With just a little oil and a lot of flavors, this dish is healthy and mouth-watering all at the same time.

This recipe needs 5-10 minutes of prep and 45 minutes of cooking. It will make four helpings.

- Fat – 38.2 g
- Protein – 31.9 g
- Net Carbs – 53.1 g
- Calories – 680

What to Use:

- For the Rice:
  - Wild Rice (0.33 cup)

- o Butter (2 tablespoons)
  - o Onion (0.5 medium-sized, chopped)
  - o White Rice (0.5 cup)
  - o Vegetable or Chicken Broth (1.25 cups)
  - o Thyme (1 teaspoon, fresh & minced)
  - o Pecans (10-12 pieces, chopped roughly)
  - o Cranberries (0.33 cup, dried)
- For the Salmon:
  - o Salmon (4-5 ounce filets)
  - o Orange Juice (0.33 cup)
  - o Butter (2 tablespoons, melted)
  - o Salt & Pepper (to taste)
  - o Thyme (1 teaspoon, fresh & minced)

What to Do:

- Preheat the oven at 425 degrees first and prepare your wild rice first.
- In a small pot, add 1.5 cups of water and your wild rice alone. Boil about 20 minutes until firm yet tender. Drain and set aside.
- Now, place the salmon on a baking dish either sprayed or lined with parchment paper. Over the salmon, pour your orange juice and melted butter, then season with salt, pepper, and thyme. Bake 15 minutes, until fully cooked.
- Once that goes in the oven, melt the rice butter in a medium pot. At medium heat, add the onion and cook 5 minutes. Then, add your rice, broth, thyme, cranberries, and pecans. Stir together and add the separated wild rice too. Bring to a boil.
- Cover and reduce to simmer, cook 15-20 minutes or until tender enough to eat. Serve with the salmon and enjoy!

Hearty Vegetable Stew

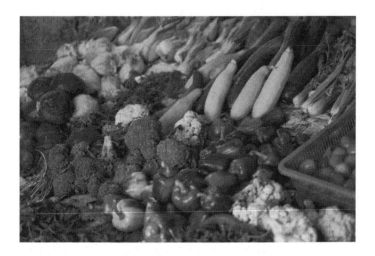

Nothing's better than throwing some veggies and broth into a pot, spicing it up, and ending up with a perfect cold-weather soup, and that's exactly what this recipe is all about. Alter the veggies as needed to incorporate the healing you desire.

This recipe needs 20 minutes of prep and 1 hour and 30 minutes of cooking. It will make 12 helpings.

- Fat – 5.9 g
- Protein – 36.5 g
- Net Carbs – 148.1 g
- Calories – 806

What to Use:

- Onion (1 small-sized, minced)
- Garlic (1 clove, minced)
- Celery (1 stalk, minced)
- Carrot (1 medium-sized, minced)
- Vegetable or Chicken Broth (0.25 cup)

- Onion (1 large-sized, chopped)
- Button Mushrooms (8 ounces, sliced)
- Portobello Mushrooms (8 ounces, sliced)
- Dried Rosemary (1 teaspoon)
- Italian Seasoning (1 teaspoon)
- Red Wine (0.5 cup)
- Vegetable or Chicken Broth (3 cups)
- Salt (0.5 teaspoon)
- Pepper (0.25 teaspoon)
- Diced Tomatoes (1-15 ounce can)
- Carrots (2 medium-sized, chopped)
- Celery (2 stalks, chopped)
- Potatoes (2 large-sized, chopped)
- Tomato Sauce (1-8 ounce can)
- Balsamic Vinegar (1 tablespoon)
- Cornstarch (1 tablespoon)
- Peas (1 cup, frozen)

What to Do:

- Prepare your minced vegetables and sauté them in a large pot with the quarter-cup of vegetable or chicken broth. Cook until softened.
- Add large-sized chopped onion and cook a while longer.
- Add mushrooms, rosemary, and Italian seasoning, and cook until liquid largely evaporates from the pan.
- Deglaze with red wine and then add the rest of the broth.
- Add tomatoes and tomato sauce as well before putting in the rest of your chopped vegetables. Turn up the heat to high and bring to boil.
- Add remaining spices and vegetables aside from cornstarch and heat through.
- Turn heat to low once peas and potatoes are cooked.

- Separately, mix cornstarch with a tablespoon of cold water until a paste is made and stir into the soup to thicken. Simmer until consistency desired is reached then enjoy!

Chicken Breast with Grilled & Raw Vegetables

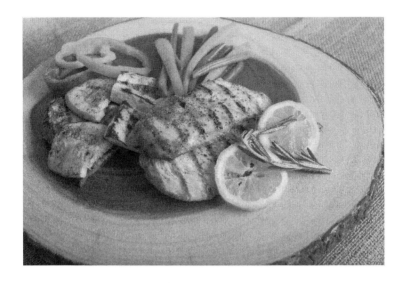

For some basic protein and vegetable, try this recipe on for size. It's incredibly simple and provides everything your body needs all in one sitting.

This recipe needs 40 minutes of prep and 20 minutes of cooking. It will make 4 helpings.

- Fat – 12.6 g
- Protein – 36.4 g
- Net Carbs – 10.4 g
- Calories – 228

What to Use:

- Chicken Breast (4 individual breasts)
- Yellow Squash (1 large-sized, trimmed & cut length-wise)
- Red Peppers (2 large-sized, deseeded & cut into large pieces)
- Marinade:

- o Olive Oil (3 tablespoons)
- o Soy Sauce (3 tablespoons)
- o Dry Mustard (2 teaspoons)
- o Balsamic Vinegar (3 tablespoons)
- o Worcestershire Sauce (2 tablespoons)
- o Garlic (2 cloves, minced)
- o Lemon Juice (2 tablespoons)
- o Salt (0.25 teaspoon)
- o Parsley (4 tablespoons, fresh & chopped)
- Celery (1 pound, cut into sticks)
- Carrots (1 pound, cut into sticks)

What to Do:

- In a small bowl, whisk the ingredients for the marinade together. Set aside.
- Prepare all the vegetables by cutting them to size, and then grab two plastic baggies.
- In one bag, pour about 2/3 of the marinade and add the chicken. Close the bag. In the other, pour the remaining third of marinade and add your veggies.
- Let marinating foods sit with sauce for about 30 minutes.
- Turn on the grill. When foods are done marinating, add the chicken breasts first. Grill about 7 minutes per side, flipping just once. Then grill the veggies, just about 3 minutes per side, flipping once.
- Serve some chicken with an even mix of raw and cooked vegetables.

Dessert Recipes

Low-Fat Blueberry Crumble

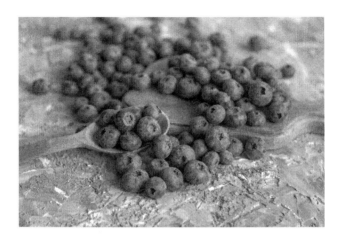

Blueberries are incredible for health, and in this low-fat dessert, you should have more than you ever wanted.

This recipe needs 20 minutes of prep and 55 minutes of baking. It will make 8 helpings.

- Fat – 8.1 g
- Protein – 2.2 g
- Net Carbs – 15 mg
- Calories – 217

What to Use:

- Cornstarch (4 teaspoons)
- Brown Sugar (2 tablespoons)
- Vanilla Extract (0.5 teaspoon)
- Blueberries (1 pound, frozen or fresh)
- Flour (0.5 cup)
- Brown Sugar (0.5 cup, packed)

- Rolled Oats (0.25 cup)
- Walnuts (3 tablespoons, chopped)
- Cornmeal (2 tablespoons)
- Salt (0.5 teaspoon)
- Cinnamon (0.25 teaspoon)
- Butter (0.25 cup, chilled & diced)

What to Do:

- Preheat the oven at 375 degrees and take a baking pan for your crumble. 8-inch square pans work well. When you have your pan, spray it with nonstick baking spray. Then sprinkle two teaspoons of the cornstarch into the pan and coat the inside with it.
- With the other two teaspoons, combine into a large bowl with two tablespoons of brown sugar, vanilla, and blueberries. Pour into the baking dish when tossed to coat.
- Combine the flour with the following six ingredients into a food processor. To combine ingredients appropriately, pulse twice. Add the butter and pulse give more times. You want this mixture to look coarse and gritty when it's "done."
- Spoon over blueberries, pack down, then bake for 30 minutes.

IF-Friendly Brownies

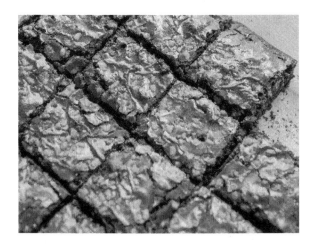

These brownies will provide that punch of sweetness without overdosing you, and it also contains coffee for an additional surge of energy afterward.

This recipe needs 5-10 minutes of prep and 30 minutes of baking. It will make 6 helpings.

- Fat – 9.7 g
- Protein – 4.6 g
- Net Carbs – 31.3 g
- Calories – 214

What to Use:

- Coffee (1 teaspoon, ground)
- Vanilla Extract (2 teaspoons)
- Oats (0.25 cup)
- Cocoa Powder (0.5 cup, unsweetened)
- Flour (0.5 cup)
- Salt (1.25 teaspoons)

- Baking Powder (0.25 teaspoon)
- Sugar (0.5 cup)
- Extra Virgin Olive Oil (0.25 cup)
- Egg Whites (3 large-sized, whites kept & separated from yolks)

What to Do:

- Preheat the oven at 350 degrees and take a baking pan for your brownies. 8-inch square pans work well. When you have your pan, spray it with nonstick baking spray.
- Take a cup and dissolve the coffee grounds into the vanilla extract. In a small bowl, mix cocoa, salt, flour, oats, and baking powder. In a larger bowl, combine sugar, oil, and egg whites. Add coffee mixture to wet mix eventually.
- Add dry mix to wet mix and blend well. Spread into the pan and bake for 20-25 minutes until a knife inserted in the middle comes out clean.
- Cool for up to two hours before eating.

Conclusion

As we come to the end of *Intermittent Fasting for Women*, I just want to thank you for making it all the way to this point! Thank you also for joining me on this adventure, for staying through till the thick of it, and for coming all the way to the end. Now, the journey turns over into your hands.

From this point further, you'll be responsible for what happens in your life about intermittent fasting. All the information you've gathered has led up to this point where you're forced to decide: Is it time for your first IF? And if not now, when? Overall, the next step involves making decisions and taking action.

I sincerely hope that my passion for health and fitness translated well for you and that you received all the information you hoped to through this book. If you've found the information in these pages useful and productive in any way, feel free to give it a review on Amazon. It's always good to know what's helpful, what works and what doesn't, and although I put lots of love and care into this text, there's always room to grow.

Thank you again for the download. Please do let me know what you think of the book! And when it comes to your personal journey with intermittent fasting, good luck and happy healing!

Made in the USA
San Bernardino, CA
21 June 2019